my mother
My Child

a caregiving daughter

shares her emotional

eight year journey.

SUSIE KINSLOW ADAMS

TATE PUBLISHING, LLC

Published in the United States of America
by Tate Publishing, LLC
127 East Trade Center Terrace
Mustang, OK 73064
(888) 361–9473

Scripture quotations marked "KJV" are taken from the
Holy Bible, King James Version, Cambridge, 1769.

Scripture quotations marked "TLB" are taken from *The
Living Bible* / Kenneth N. Taylor: Tyndale House, ©
Copyright 1997, 1971 by Tyndale House Publishers, Inc.
Used by permission. All rights reserved.

This book is designed to provide accurate and authorita-
tive information with regard to the subject matter covered.
This information is given with the understanding that
neither the author nor Tate Publishing, LLC is engaged
in rendering legal, professional advice. Since the details
of your situation are fact dependent, you should addition-
ally seek the services of a competent professional.

ISBN: 1–5988623-8-3

DEDICATION

This book is dedicated to my husband,
Russell, whose love, compassion, and
understanding never wavered;

To my brother, Richard, who faithfully
called his mother every Saturday night
for thirty years, and who continues to call
me at least once every week;

And to God whose grace has proven
sufficient. To Him be all honor
and praise.

ACKNOWLEDGEMENTS

*B*efore the first word was penned, seven women agreed to pray daily for God to guide and direct each step of the way. I am eternally indebted to Laura Adams, Judy Divine, Linda Erickson, Edna Mitchell, Sue Walter, Sheri White, and Sharon Williams, for their faithfulness and support. Four of my prayer partners also spent endless hours reading and re-reading the manuscript: Laura, Judy, Linda, and Sue. I appreciate your honesty (and bravery) in keeping me on target; your input proved invaluable.

For the Dallas County pastors and their wives and so many others who not only prayed, but also nudged me to continue when the way got rough, I am deeply humbled and grateful.

I am sincerely thankful for the physicians and healthcare workers who shared valuable time to review portions of the manuscript.

It has been a joy to work with Tate Publishing. Your confidence in this venture has been demonstrated by your exceptional staff, and their untiring efforts to see it to completion.

TABLE OF CONTENTS

FOREWORD

↵

"This is an important book. It *needs* to be written." I clearly remember my reaction when I read the first few pages my mom had penned. Until reading those lines that gave birth to this book, I had no idea what my mother had experienced during the eight years that she cared for my Grandma. All I knew was that my mom was too busy to get on a plane and come visit me. I had no concept of the long hours she worked, the life and death decisions she had to make and the emotional and physical turmoil she faced daily. I had no idea because she never once complained or let on that providing full time care for my Grandma was difficult work. My mom truly cherished each and every moment of caring for her mother.

In life and in this book my mom has taught me that to love another means being committed to providing the very best possible for them, regardless of one's personal sacrifice. The story that she shares in this book demonstrates that while caring for an ailing loved one's physical needs is important, enveloping them with affection, affirmation and encouragement brings even deeper healing, healing of the heart, healing for the one receiving care and the one giving care. I am confident that in these pages, you too will learn from my mom's strong, loving, selfless example.

Laura Adams
Founder, Photo Legacy Project

INTRODUCTION

⌒

"Surely I will never have to take care of my
mother when she gets old. Can you imagine
what she will be like? She is so independent and quick
tempered. She will be a real challenge for anyone to
care for. I couldn't do it, I just couldn't do it. I wouldn't
even try!"

How clearly those words rang in my ears as
I stood over Mother's bed, not knowing if she would
live or die. We had taken her to the emergency room
after she suddenly began hemorrhaging and she was
immediately admitted to the hospital. Mother had
congestive heart failure and her overall health was not
good. She did not seem to have the strength or the
will to fight this latest battle. The doctors said that she
had continued to weaken, and I should prepare for the
worst.

As I watched what had been such a strong-willed person seem to wilt before my eyes, my whole being just wanted to swoop her up into my arms and rock her gently as she did me so many times. Mother was loving and nurturing, always giving generously to her family and friends. Never once had I heard harmful words come from her mouth as she faithfully cared for her aging parents and so many others.

Tears flowed freely as I stroked her brow and thought of those hurtful words and how carelessly I had uttered them. Warm drops fell on her face as I kissed her cheeks. She was entirely helpless and completely dependent on those around her for care. How could her only daughter ever have had such feelings or dare express them to someone else.

My heart broke again and again as I prayed. "Lord, please forgive me for ever saying such a thing about her. Forgive me for my selfish attitude and my uncaring ways. And, Heavenly Father, if You just let her live, I promise to care for her with all I have for as long as it takes until You see fit to take her home."

Week after week, I spent many hours in prayer receiving God's forgiveness and begging Him in His grace to allow us some time together. This was all too sudden and I was unprepared to let her go. Night and day I was at Mother's bedside, holding her hand, stroking her forehead, and kissing her cheek. Tears flowed freely and often as I recounted precious memories from days gone by.

My husband, Russell, and I had lived in California for ten years. Our short annual trips home had offered little time to spend with my mother. Now, after moving back to Missouri and living just two hours away from Mother, I thought we would finally be able to make up for lost time. Perhaps we could go sightseeing and shopping; maybe out to eat and once again enjoy great times together. Watching her struggle in this hospital for her very life was not a part of my plan. Hopes and dreams shattered as life suddenly changed for all of us in ways we could not imagine.

God was merciful; after seven long weeks of ups and downs, Mother was released from the hospital and came to live with us for eight wonderful years. This book is about those years and the trials and triumphs of caring for her through the many changes that ensued. It's about those tender truths God taught me about myself as He and I journeyed together.

This book is not meant to be an instruction manual to help in caring for someone. There are volumes available on the practical aspects of elder care. This book is an opportunity for me to relate openly and honestly the struggles and the victories of life with a parent who suddenly becomes your child. My intent is simply to share my heart in hopes that others may relate and perhaps be helped by knowing they are not in this alone.

MIRACLES, MOVES, AND MOTHER

*M*y mother has always held a special place in my heart. She had a rough life but made the best of it. She worked hard and seldom complained about anything, although there was much opportunity to do so. During the years that I lived by Mother, especially after Dad died, we would spend time going out to eat or visiting some beautiful scenic place not too far from home. One of my fondest memories is of her and me sitting on her front porch enjoying the soft breeze and breathing in the crisp morning air.

"How could anyone ever look out at God's creation and not know He is real?" she would ask. Then she would continue to elaborate on the beauty of her surroundings. An outsider driving by would only see shabby yards and small homes in need of major repair, and would probably complain at the rough streets. But my mother could see the good neighbors and the beautiful flowers among the weeds. She was thankful for her comfortable home and the reliability of her very old automobile parked out front.

Mother had a sharp mind and a quick wit. She was always ready with an answer for any problem one might have (and quite sure that hers was the only answer to consider). Her tiny home was always clean and orderly; you could count on a good pot of stew and cornbread when you stopped by for a visit.

After Russell and I moved away, I especially looked forward to coming back home to those familiar sights and sounds and that hearty welcome from someone who dearly loved me. During the ten years that we were in California, my visits were short and too far apart. However I never worried about Mother's well-being because she was active in a good church, a Bible study group, and had several other widowed friends with whom to socialize. On the surface she seemed quite self sufficient.

I never noticed when she got old and weary; when she quit caring for her little home and herself as she once did. When I began to realize how terribly unclean her house was, I attributed it to her being too busy to keep it up. One year I made a planned trip home without Russell. I had thought if I could thoroughly clean her house for her, maybe she would be able to keep it clean. I know how it is when you get so far behind that it seems impossible to ever catch up. As I set out to clean Mother's home, my cleaning stopped abruptly when I was told, "This house is clean enough for me. If it is not clean enough for you, you can just go home!" Ouch!

I must admit, I think my focus was more on the unclean house than on why my mother would let it get that way. What was happening to her? Could I have done something to help her then? Perhaps get some help in each week or even check with her doctor concerning her medications? But my visit was short; whatever I could do in a week's time would not make much of a difference in the over all picture.

The day before I was to head back to California, I drove Mother to the store in her old but faithful car. As we neared home, we were stopped by the police. He announced that "my" tags were expired. After learning that I was driving Mother's car, he asked for her driver's license and registration. When she couldn't seem to find her license, the officer told us to go straight home and park the car. Back home we searched the unending piles of mail and papers on her tables and found an expired license. Wanting to help, I took Mother to take a test and get her license renewed only to find out that she had lost her license due to too many traffic tickets. No driver's license, no tags, and no insurance, yet she was still driving her car all over town.

Something wasn't right but I had a plane to catch in the morning. What could I do at this point? How could I help her? Should I alert church friends, neighbors, and the police? If I took her car keys, she would find another set or have copies made. Anything I could have done would simply be a temporary fix until I got out of town when she would do as she pleased anyway. My heart ached as I thought of leaving. How helpless I felt.

My heart and mind were eased somewhat knowing that my cousin Penny checked on Mother every few days to make sure she was okay. Penny would bring Mother back to her home when she could coax her into it. Penny would trim her nails, wash her hair, and stuff her full of good food and special treats. Mother enjoyed those times, but she always pressed to get back to her own home.

One time when Penny was traveling out west, she had a persistent feeling she should come home early from her trip. Those urgings became so overwhelming that she had her flight changed and returned to Missouri a week early. She immediately called Mother and was relieved to hear that familiar happy voice assuring her that she was okay. In fact, Mother had a Bible study planned the next day at her house, and had been very busy with all the preparations.

The following evening Penny was not too alarmed when Mother didn't answer her phone. "Perhaps," she thought, "Aunt Nevie has just gone to the store for something." However, when there was no response the second day, Penny was on Mother's doorstep. Unlocking the door, she found Mother on the floor, somewhat dehydrated.

Apparently, after the Bible study group had left, Mother sat down to rest on a low sofa instead of her usual recliner. She was short, quite heavy, and not as agile as she had thought. Realizing she could not get up from the couch on her own, Mother slid onto the floor. She was sure she would then be able turn around and pull herself up. Once on the floor though, she had neither the strength nor the mobility to get up on her own.

"Aunt Nevie, why didn't you call someone when you couldn't get up by yourself?"

"I would have called if I needed help. I was going to get up soon." In her mind, all she needed to do was rest a spell and try again. Eventually, she reasoned, she would be able to get up from that floor.

What would have happened if no one had checked on her? What if Penny hadn't followed the tug of her heart to come home early? Did God bring Penny back home just in time to help her Aunt Nevie? She is convinced He did, and so am I.

It was just a short time later that Russell was called as Pastor of the First Baptist Church of Fair Play, Missouri and we moved back home. A few weeks after our move, Penny brought Mother to visit us and we would again see God's timing. It was during that visit that Mother became hospitalized for the first time, and our lives would change forever. For eight years I would be the primary caregiver for my Mother and, although I didn't realize it then, would watch her slip into what we often call "second childhood." Some of those years Mother communicated normally and was up and around even fixing her own lunch. Other times she would not be able to walk without help or carry on a conversation.

Mother's life, too, changed drastically. She found herself living with her children in a strange new house and in a town that she couldn't locate on the map. Everyone who came in and out of the house was a stranger to her. Gone were the days of getting a hamburger with old friends after Bible Study. Gone was her freedom to go anywhere by herself or just pick up the phone and call a neighbor to come over. Only in looking back now do I recognize how very, very different life had become for Mother as well as for Russell and me.

Growing up, our home was always pleasant, comfortable, and full of love, yet the boundaries were clearly marked. Dad, Richard and I never pried into Mother's affairs. As an adult, I knew a few details concerning where certain papers were kept should they be needed, but asking for more information was sure to bring a clear expression that it was actually none of my business. Discussing Mother's financial well-being was clearly out of the question.

Have you ever watched children raiding Mom or Grandma's purse for candy or gum? I've seen all ages, even Dads, digging through a woman's purse looking for something they needed or wanted. What a difference it was with my Mother's generation. You did not raid Mother's purse; you didn't even pick it up or look as though you were going to touch it. That purse contained her personal belongings and was not for anyone, not even her husband, to explore.

When I began to accept the fact that Mother really was not stable mentally, I knew it was up to me to look at her checkbook and bills to determine where she was financially. After she had gone to bed one night, I took her purse into my bedroom and just held it. I felt like a criminal getting ready to rob someone. I was betraying my own mother by going through her personal belongings. It is difficult to explain the trauma of such a seemingly small task. As I considered simply approaching her about her finances, the old fears of the past would rise up. I could hear her telling me to mind my own business. Here I was with kids and grandkids of my own, still afraid of the wrath of Momma. It took nearly an hour for me to open her purse that night.

Those feelings of betrayal surfaced again when I had to explain to Mom the need for me to be on her checking account so I could purchase her medicines and pay her doctor as well as her utilities until she could go back to her own home. Amazingly, the changes were made easily with only smiles of approval from Mother (Was God at it again?). In the beginning, I kept Mother's purse by her chair and let her give me the checkbook when I needed it, always making sure to tell her what I bought or what had been paid from her account. It was important that she have plenty of cash in her wallet so she could have access to spending money and feel in control of her finances. She was proud to offer to pay for lunch when we were taking her out to the doctor's office, or to be able to buy something from kids who came by selling their wares. I'm sure that she did not understand all that was happening but having cash on hand seemed to make her feel secure, more independent and a real part of the decision making process. How difficult it must be on adults when they begin to realize they are no longer responsible enough to handle their own affairs.

Russell and I talked at length about Mother's care. We both agreed from the very first that she would be in our home as long as we could care for her no matter what it cost in time, money, or personal convenience. Putting her in a nursing home was not an option for us unless we were convinced that would be in her best interest.

During Mother's first hospital stay, many decisions had to be made quickly. A caring nurse helped Mother understand the importance of being prepared for these occasions, and encouraged her to sign papers appointing me as her power of attorney in health care matters. By slowly and carefully going over each option, Mother was able to make good choices on her own about what she wanted done in each situation. This step became even more beneficial as time went on and decisions became more immediate and increasingly critical.

I feel it is necessary to note here that it is vitally important that life and death decisions be made as early as possible before emotions get in the way, and while a person has the reasoning to make them. Had we waited much longer, Mother would not have had the presence of mind to make those important choices. Without a Durable Power of Attorney and Health Care Directive, it would have been much more difficult to determine her wishes as we took care of her. Even though we had to evaluate our decisions constantly to meet her ever-changing situation, a clear understanding from the beginning was invaluable.

We must be prepared for unexpected events that can change our lives drastically *regardless of our age or our circumstances.* When Mother closed her front door to go on what she had thought would be just a short trip, she could not have realized that she would never return to her little home. In a matter of time her two children would have to make decisions concerning her home and belongings that she could no longer make for herself. I was thankful that I could legally take care of her financial and business matters. This in itself did much to free my attention to focus on her health and personal needs.

Russell and I and my brother, Richard, continually discussed options available and always kept communications open so that there were no surprises later. It was important to me that my brother review her finances with me when he visited so that he would know exactly where every penny of Mother's money was being used. He did not think it was necessary, but it gave me peace of mind. I never did get comfortable making decisions about her money.

As time passed, it became apparent to us that

Mother would not be going back to her home again. Being her only daughter, it seemed a natural duty of mine to determine what to do with all her belongings. Her home was a couple of hours away so I packed a bag and headed for Webb City. I spent several days in the house alone, some of the most difficult days of my life. Every room and every piece of furniture held memories of better days. Drawers and cabinets were packed with "stuff." Important items to my mother, I am sure; to me, just something more to store or dispose of so the house could be rented or sold. When I realized that I could not take the time to sort each paper, I purchased some large garbage bags. I dumped drawers and boxes of papers into the bags to bring home. Later, as time permitted, I could filter out the important papers, if any, and discard the rest.

In the years that have passed since I cleaned out Mother's house, I have taken inventory of my own home. We sorted and disposed of boxes full of papers and things that would mean absolutely nothing to our children. At one point, I even sorted my cabinets and kitchen drawers. Any item we were not currently using was put in a box for some agency that helped the needy in our community. Together, Russell and I made lists of important papers and where they were stored. We insisted our two boys sit down with us and listen as we told them of our insurance policies and where to find them. We also told them of our prepaid burial policies and where they were. The boys, of course, did not want to consider these issues, but it was so very important that they be informed should something happen to one or both of us.

When Mother did come home to live with us, food preparation was a big hurdle for me. She had been an extraordinary cook. She served as dinner cook for many years in a fine restaurant. At home, she could make banquets from meager supplies. Now I would be preparing all of her meals. Would she like what I fixed? Would I cook everything right? Did I know enough about what she needed to eat to do a good job of planning? I would soon learn that no matter what I prepared, she would practically inhale it to the last crumb, and we would all be healthier as a result of my wiser food choices.

It seemed that every part of Mother's life was changing overnight. She had worn slacks and pretty blouses for years, but these would no longer work. It was much easier for her to slip a dress over her head than to put on pants. Short nightgowns and pretty polyester dresses or robes seemed to be the best choice as her health waned. There were days when her clothes had to be changed three or four times. Each time I was given a choice between frustration and fun; I chose fun.

Finding clothing that fit her short, wide frame without falling off her narrow shoulders was a challenge. I am so thankful for mail order catalogues, the internet shopping venues, and an old Montgomery Ward store. I bought her the most colorful clothing I could find. Using lacy nightgowns as a slip, I matched them with simple polyester housedresses.

"You is a beautiful girl, Mommy!"

She would giggle and reply as I changed her garment, "I is a beautiful girl."

"You is a soggy girl, too!"

"Is I?"

"You is, but I loves you anyway."

"Me, too!"

As far back as I can remember, Mother always had difficulty finding good fitting shoes for her swollen ankles and feet. For the first several years that I shopped for her, I had to buy men's bedroom slippers to get the width she needed. Additional care had to be taken that any footwear not have slippery soles on them. Her slippers, like everything else she wore, had to be washable because, as I told her, she "leaked".

As she lost weight, her feet and ankles slimmed also. How exciting it was to shop for pretty ballerina slippers to match her colorful dresses. What joy to watch her hold her feet up and smile at her new shoes and slim ankles; like a little girl with her first pair of dress shoes.

Mother found it difficult to lift her short, heavy legs up into the bed on her own so we devised a system to help her. While sitting on the bed, she would put both her feet on a footstool which Russell had previously shortened for this purpose. Slowly and carefully I would then raise her legs and guide them onto the bed as she gradually reclined. As long as she had the strength to help me, I did very little actual lifting myself. With a little encouragement and direction, it was amazing what she was able to accomplish.

My fear that Mother would be lonely in her new surroundings was an entirely misguided concern. Without our asking, ladies from our church began visiting Mother, whether or not we were home. Returning one day to find a fresh bouquet of flowers on her table, I questioned her about the company she had while we were out.

"No one was here," she replied.

"No one? Who brought those beautiful flowers?"

"They were just here."

As the mother I knew began to disappear, new challenges surfaced constantly as Russell and I adjusted our lives to her changing condition. One of the more difficult things for me to reconcile was the fact that getting help meant people would be in and out of our home throughout the week. I enjoyed company; the kind that come and sit and visit or maybe eat a little something, and then go home. I was not comfortable at first with people coming in and wandering throughout our home, but I knew it was necessary for the well being of our entire family.

When neighbors, Jessie and Wilus Ahart, learned we were caring for Mother, Jessie offered to stay with her one day a week and other times as needed. She was even willing to stay overnight so we could go to a retreat or just get away. This took much pressure off when we needed to get home later than we had originally planned. We could call Jessie to come over and pull the blinds, close the door, turn up the heat or whatever was needed. Whether it was a sudden storm approaching or an uneasiness she sensed, Jessie checked on Mother as though caring for her own family. Jessie grew to love Mother right away; it showed in the way she cared for her. Jessie loved to quote the Bible and talk about the Lord. This seemed to please Mother. Often we would come home to find the two of them watching a gospel music video together.

"We've had the best visit," Jessie would say. "We've been talking about Heaven, haven't we, Geneva? And we are going there, aren't we?" Momma would smile and nod in agreement. Clearly this was a mutual admiration between the two as well as a welcomed respite for a weary caregiver.

Those four years at Fair Play were often challenging as we constantly faced new obstacles in Mother's care. Physically she would go back and forth from being strong and walking on her own to not being able to get out of her chair without help. At one point a nurse had to come every day to care for Mother's swollen legs. They were so full of fluid they had to be wrapped each day. Open wounds would redden and weep. We wondered if she would ever be able to walk on them again. With good care and her own resilience, she was soon able to move from room to room with the aid of her walker.

Personal care was a hard issue for me to deal with at first. Since my children were ten and eleven when I became their mother, I had never cared for a baby or small child. I had no skills at all in that area, and the thought of bathing my mother and caring for her was difficult to comprehend. Oh, I wanted to do it, I just didn't know how. That may sound silly to folks who have raised little ones, but for me bathing Mother was monumental.

At first, Mother seemed to be caring for herself pretty well although needing help with personal care was inevitable. I dreaded confronting her with the possibility of me helping her. I was relieved when the doctor ordered a bath aide to come out three times a week.

Mary Long was our first experience with a regularly scheduled bath aide. Right away I knew that she would be good for Mother. Watching Mary pamper Mom as she bathed her was a comfort to this worried daughter. Mother was talking and reasoning well when Mary first came so they had ample opportunity to get acquainted. They shared about their families and their likes and dislikes. By the time Mother had quit talking Mary had developed a loving relationship with her. I learned so much about how to care for my mother from Mary. I'm convinced that her good care and what she taught us kept Mom from having any bedsores or serious skin problems at home.

When Russell resigned from the church in Fair Play, we had to move out of the church parsonage. Finding a home within driving distance of Mother's doctor became a priority. Financially we felt we were not ready to buy a newer home, so we considered a fixer-upper. We soon realized that homes "needing a little repair" in our price range generally needed a demolition crew.

Our search was both fun and challenging as we considered what would be comfortable and convenient for Mother and at the same time meet our personal needs. After looking a few weeks, we were thrilled to find the home that we are sure, beyond any doubt, that God had saved just for us. The things we had wanted were all there: big picture window, large room for Mom, extra bathroom, front and back porches and trees in the yard. What we had not expected to get were extra wide doorways which would easily accommodate her wheelchair, access to the home without steps to deal with, a fireplace, an oversized shower with easy access in her bathroom, a huge walk-in closet in her area, an eat-in kitchen, a big dining room, and an acre of ground surrounded by fields and woods. Only God could know how important every one of these things would be as we faced another four years with Mom. And God knew we would not have time to remodel anything.

March 29, 2000, my calendar says "Move everything possible today." That means Momma, too. How were we actually going to be able to get all this done without added stress on her? We described our new home and encouraged her to help us decide what we should take with us. We even asked her opinion on the pictures and furniture that we should keep, all the while knowing that she wouldn't remember later. We decided to sell most of what we had in a garage sale and replace only what we needed in the new house.

Down came all the pictures from the walls. Chairs, tables, and accessories were quickly moved out as they were sold. At the same time we were moving boxes of personal items into our new home. Finally, all that was left in the church parsonage was Mother sitting alone in her wheelchair in a big, empty room with nothing but a small borrowed television set in one corner.

"Mommy, where is all our stuff? You look kind of lonesome there all by yourself in this big old room." I wondered what she was thinking as she slowly smiled at me.

"Do you think we ought to just move you, too? Shall I call for the transportation van to take you to our new home?" That wide familiar grin and nodding head told me she was ready to go anywhere we went. Someone who doesn't comprehend what is being said or is not able to retain information needs things repeated again and again. We described our new town and home so many times we tired of the telling. However, it seemed to help Mother feel part of the move and comfortable with the strange activity around her. I never ever wanted her to feel like she was an added-on part of our family or in any way a burden to us.

Watching Mother's eyes light up as she was unloaded in Buffalo was all the assurance I needed that she would be just fine with the move. Thinking she would be tired from the trip, I started to wheel her into her new bedroom, but she had other ideas. She wanted to see the entire house, into every room and through every doorway. When she had explored everything to her satisfaction, she was content to settle down in her own room for a much-needed nap.

My greatest fear in the move was losing our dear helpers, Mary and Jessie. Miraculously, God had worked this dilemma out as well. One day while still in the old house, Mary came in with the saddest look on her face. She told us that most of her work would now be in Dallas County; Mother was actually her last client in Polk County. At the same time that we had been dreading the thoughts of telling Mary of our move, she had been hesitant to tell us that she could no longer come to Fair Play. What joy to say, "Mary, we are moving to Dallas County, too!"

When Jessie and Wilus heard about our new home, they were actually excited. Jessie said, "That is just a good forty-five minute trip for us. We will look forward to the drive to the country. Call us anytime you need help." Wow! They were happy! We were happy! Mom was still in good care! And God had again proven to be faithful far beyond my wildest dreams!

Three months after we moved, Russell was called as Director of Missions of the Dallas County Association of Southern Baptists. Retirement was short-lived and we were on a new journey. And, so was Mother. Little did we know what an adventure it would be for all of us, and how good it would be for her. She would get more attention and love than ever, and we would come to know more than we ever wanted about caring for the elderly and the truths of what we call second childhood.

Mother's stepfather and mother,
Oscar and Louella Doke.

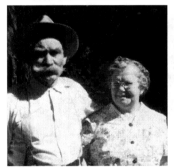

Grandma Doke and daughters
Geneva and Josephine

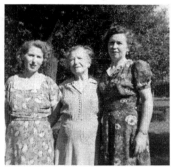

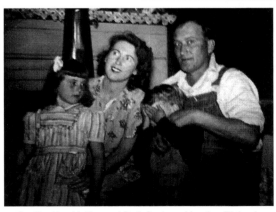

Our Family - Mother and Dad, Susie and brother Richard

Frank

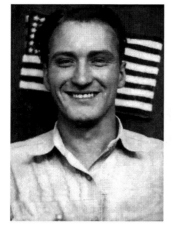

Geneva

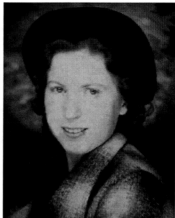

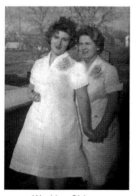

Working Girls -
Susie and Mother

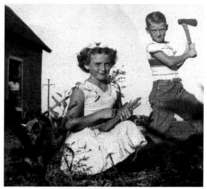

Susie and Richard

WHERE ARE YOU, MOMMA?

～

"*I* don't know who you are, but you are not my daughter!"

I can still to this day hear the words and see the expression on her face. As I dressed Mom and combed her hair I had said something to her about being glad she was with us. Somewhere in the conversation when I had called her "Mother," she interrupted me. Not harsh words at all, but very, very firm and confident.

The words stung at my very soul and I wanted to run and cry, to flee somewhere for some solitude. But it was not to be. I had to continue my work and help her be comfortable with this now strange woman caring for her.

She continued, "I am not your mother."

Only God could have gotten me through that one!

"Well, you are somebody's mother, aren't you?"

"I is."

"I am sure you are a very, very special mother. Is it okay if I just call you Mom? I sure would like that."

"Okay, if you want to."

"I love you, pretty lady. You are very sweet, and loving, too!"

She smiled broadly in approval as we slowly made our way into the living room for breakfast.

The tears flowed later as I sat on the back deck thinking how much I missed her. She never said those words again to me but I often wondered if she really knew who I was or whether I was just some nice person caring for her.

I have heard people trying to convince someone who they were in these circumstances and I am sure there is a time when that is appropriate. I did not think it was as important for her to know me as it was for her to know that she was well, safe, and getting good care. This had to be the priority. I could and would adjust to anything. She, on the other hand, was pretty fragile in her thinking and didn't need the added stress.

We have all made jokes about second childhood, blaming our lack of memory or energy on it. Older folk do seem to forget more and aren't as productive as they once were. We've laughed at the possibility of going back to no teeth, no hair, and diapers. In reality, watching your own mother actually reach these stages is not a laughing matter. As my mother became more child-like in her thinking and her actions, by necessity I would take on a parent-like role. She would need more personalized attention. She had to be watched like a young child so that she didn't hurt herself with something. It became a mixed blessing that she could no longer get out of a chair without help; at least she couldn't wander off or suffer a fall.

But she was still my mother and she needed to be reminded often. Or, was it I who needed the reminder from time to time? I called her Mother. I sought her advice. I sought her approval in whatever I was doing. I respected her position as mother, while caring for her as a child. She was now as dependent on me as I had been on her as a baby.

Two days before Christmas 1998, Mother had cancer cells removed from her nose. My once strong I-can-face-anything Mother looked so frightened when she was being prepared for surgery. She held onto a straw all the time she was in the hospital, and the nurses let her keep it going into surgery. When I saw her in the recovery room, I was surprised to find she still had that straw in her hand. Like a child's favorite toy or blankie buys comfort in strange situations, that familiar object in Mother's hand gave her courage to face yet another new experience.

She came home from the operation with a big ball of cotton gauze attached to the end of her nose. I was given strict instructions to not let her touch it. Right! What would you do if you peered down your nose and saw a big cotton ball on the end of it? It was difficult at times but she did a pretty good job of leaving the bandage alone (at least while we were watching).

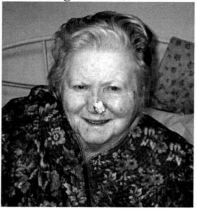

When the stitches were removed the Doctor said her nose would be red for months, and I was to keep her hands away from it. The scab kept coming off. Was this normal? Was she pulling the scab off when we weren't watching? Was the skin damaged? Would it grow back? Should I call the doctor knowing the difficulty of transporting her if he wanted her to come into the office? There was no excess redness; no streaks anywhere and apparently no soreness. She looked up at me with such child-like trust, that cute smile and twinkling eyes. I could only pray: "Lord, into Your capable, trustworthy, loving, caring hands I commit my precious Momma and me, the best I know how."

Every night I cared for Mom's nose, cleaning it carefully with antiseptic wash just as the doctor had ordered before I tucked her into bed.

"Momma, don't touch your nose."

"I ain't gonna touch my nose!"

Long after she should have been sound asleep I walked into her room just in time to see her little fingers feeling that nose, busy as can be.

"Momma, whatcha doing?"

Ever bit the little girl, she quickly tucked those nimble fingers under the covers, "I ain't touched it! I didn't! I ain't gonna touch it!"

I just smiled, gave her a hug and a kiss and a silent prayer. "She's Yours, Lord. Care for her real good!"

The nose would heal eventually, and yes, the skin would be white because she had picked off the scab. But I did not care; it still functioned just fine, and she was happy! Again, I would be reminded that there are many things not worth arguing or fretting over. Life is way too short and too precious to care whether or not you have a white spot on the end of your nose!

About the time I would think I had all the answers, a new challenge would surface. Many had to do with health issues, and I was fortunate to have patient doctors and nurses to help with those as they arose. While some seemed insignificant on the surface, if they affected Mother's day-to-day routine or her peace of mind, they became extremely important to me.

I was not content to have her sitting around with absolutely nothing to do with her hands. It was difficult, however, to find things to keep her occupied, even briefly. A short-term solution arrived quite unexpectedly when we brought home tiny bottles of bubbles from a friend's wedding. Mother was so happy with her latest adventure that Russell later bought her a larger bottle of bubbles. Like a child with a new toy, she was elated! As I watched Russell trying to read with bubbles floating all around him, I wondered if he ever questioned that purchase. I wondered, too, if those bubbles "just happened" to float his way, or was someone's orneriness showing!

The deep love my husband and my mother shared was evident in the way they communicated

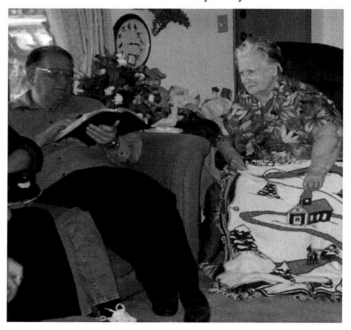

with one another. Often she would stare at him until he looked at her. A smile from him, and she was quite content. It was almost as if she were seeking his approval.

He enjoyed teasing her, and she had her way of getting back at him when least expected. During one hospital stay, he was doing his best to encourage her to

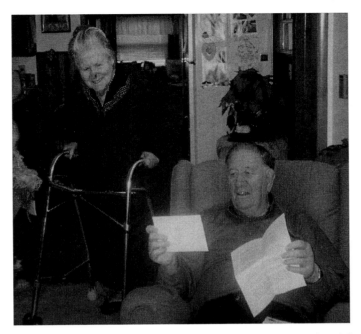

eat. "Just look at that great food," he said. "You should eat some of it. It sure looks good!"

My spunky mother replied quickly. "If it looks so good to you, then you eat it."

Mother loved books and magazines with pictures so I always left material on her table to enjoy. By the time I realized she was chewing on them, she had completely riddled the back of a magazine. What could I do? I didn't want to take everything away from her and leave her with nothing to challenge her thinking.

Small children's books with thick pages were easy for her to handle and not as easy to tear up. She really enjoyed holding them and could read the big print easily. This was the answer to our dilemma. However, as with most things, this was only a temporary solution. When she began chewing the pages again, it was time to go shopping once more.

I found what was needed for our current crisis in the baby department; a book with padded cloth pages, rubber corners and plastic teething rings on the binder. It was very colorful, washable, and actually made to be chewed on. I was going to purchase an infant's book for my mother!

I bought the book, but I couldn't give it to her. I looked at the book, looked at my mother, and it just didn't seem to fit. I laid the book aside for several days; I could not hand it to her. When her chewing persisted and I took the other books and cards away, she seemed to miss them so much. One day I just put the new book on the edge of her table while I was moving some things around in her room. Then as I cleared her food tray, I left the book there. I was later relieved to see her chewing on the plastic corners and looking through the thick, fabric pages.

"Isn't that a neat little book? Should I leave it here awhile?"

Her expression said, "Yes." We had met the latest challenge and had yet another look at the child within. My emotions ran wild each time we crossed another hurdle. I was so happy to have found something to meet her present needs. At the same time I was hurt and torn inside to watch my beautiful mother so content to chew and drool all over a child's toy.

I've scarcely had to care for anyone who had more than a cold or flu, or ever had any long-term illnesses myself. As children, we seldom went to a doctor; Mother always seemed to know what to do to care for us. Now, I could no longer depend upon her wisdom. She was in my care going from one predicament to another, almost daily, and I had to make tough decisions all alone. I didn't know how to make everything better for her. I soon learned that if I wasn't nervous, she wouldn't be either. We made every doctor's visit a journey and every new medicine a celebration. Russell and I always did a lot of kidding with her. Mother would giggle a lot, and seemed to take most changes in stride.

Whenever Russell had to take any medicine, he was careful to take it exactly as prescribed. If he was supposed to take a pill in the morning, it was at the same exact time each day. Not so with me! I never had to take much medicine, and when I did, I took it whenever it was convenient. I generally plopped my one pill a day into my mouth some time between arising and lunch with a glass of water, and that was it for the day.

Now however, I had my mother's health and well-being in my hands. She would take whatever I handed her; I had to be sure medicines were given correctly and on time. I needed to pay closer attention to details: take with fluids; take before meals, after meals, with meals; crush, don't crush. Her prescriptions were constantly changing and it was up to me to keep abreast of the situation. In the beginning, after I had filled her weekly pillbox, I would check it again and again to be sure I had made no mistakes. About the time I got really comfortable with the schedule of her medicines, she decided she would eat them like candy. There was absolutely no way she was going to swallow her pills without chewing them first. Some of them I would be able to pulverize but not gel caps and the like.

This presented two distinct challenges to contend with. I had to notify the pharmacy or the physician that the pill would be chewed up whether or not it was supposed to be. Often the pharmacist would have a liquid or a smaller, more manageable dose that could be substituted. The next challenge was to check Mother's mouth every time she took medicines to make sure there were no pills tucked away in her cheeks or under her tongue.

I had always checked for the availability of generics when a new prescription was ordered from the pharmacy. One day I decided to inquire about generics for her older prescriptions as well. Mother had been paying $103.00 a month for Vasotec. By calling her pharmacist, I learned a generic had been released at a cost of $22.00. By taking time to make one simple phone call, I had saved her over eighty dollars a month on this one prescription. From that time on, I called the pharmacy every four or five months to inquire about the latest available generics.

Flu bugs and colds are always a concern, especially with children and the elderly and Mother all of a sudden seemed to fit into both categories. On her 89ᵗʰ birthday, she came down with a virus or flu with deep, deep congestion and fever. She stared blankly at us when we tried to talk to her. Those once sharp blue eyes now reflected a sad, worried, very sick child looking for someone to make it better. The first dose of antibiotics the doctor sent had to be literally washed down her; by the second dose, she was chewing it up and swallowing it. But I will never forget that faint, faint smile as she began to mend again.

It was difficult to know when to call a doctor because sometimes the medicine was harder on her than the illness we were treating. An allergic reaction to one medicine suddenly turned her beet red. The doctor had me immediately stop giving it to her. When she continued to redden, a visit to the emergency room was in order. New medicines were prescribed and she was soon back home again. But her skin began to peel and we had loose skin to contend with for days.

"Mommy, you is peelin'! You is gonna' be a new woman one of these days!"

Her laughter was enough to ease my worries. This little girl was going to make it again.

I placed a comfortable chair next to Mother's recliner in our living room so I could sit close and hold her soft little hand or help her with her food. She always seemed to enjoy watching me as I put curlers in my hair. One night I asked her, "Mommy, would you consider finishing my hair for me? I am tired!" What an expression she gave me as I continued, "You could do it! You used to curl my hair when I was small and you did a good job. Please?"

She just giggled and looked sweet while her looks let me know the truth of the situation: "You are a funny girl. There is no way I am helping you."

The mother I remember would have been over there doing my hair in a minute. She used to work six or seven days in a row in a hot kitchen and come home exhausted. Yet she always had time to give me permanents. She even did hair for my girlfriends and their mothers. That she did after fixing a large hot meal for her family with biscuits and gravy, home-canned vegetables, and delicious casseroles. I know she took care of my needs when her feet hurt and she ached to just sit and rest awhile. Now I could remind her of those days, and thank her once again.

"Mother, thank you for all the times you did my hair for me. You always made me look so pretty. I love you." Once more I asked the Lord to help me always be there for her as she was for me; regardless of how tired or busy I seemed to be.

As Mother became more dependent, she seldom began any conversation or gave hugs on her own. Those times she did are etched permanently in my memory. Every morning I would sit her up on the edge of her bed, put my arm around her and give her big hugs. One such morning she slowly moved her hand over my blouse and rested it on my chest. She seemed to melt onto my shoulder like a baby does when held. Those rare times were so precious, it was impossible for me to move and end the moment. As I kissed her forehead and nuzzled her a little, it's the familiar smells of my childhood that reminded me that this is still my Mother. I rejoiced and yet the lonely child's heart inside of me was breaking in two.

She often watched Russell and me as if wanting to communicate. From Russell, a simple smile or word would do. When she stared at me, she usually wanted something. It became my task to figure out what she needed.

"Need to go to the bathroom, Mom?" She continued to stare and slightly smile.

"Cold?" Same response.

"Momma, are you hungry?" Big smile!

It was refreshing to catch her staring at me occasionally with a definite sense of approval in her eyes. I wondered what she was thinking. Was she saying, "I love you, too," in the only way she could? I hoped that was the case.

About the time I would think she was merely parroting what we said to her and not really thinking at all, she would surprise us with some conversation clearly her own. I wondered how much is up there that she didn't see any reason to verbalize. She was never one for small talk anyway and she may have just gotten tired of our day-to-day silliness.

"Howdy!"

"Howdy," Mother echoed as I sat her up on the edge of her bed.

"Well, aren't you just a bundle of joy this morning?"

She mirrored my words, "Aren't you just a bundle of joy this morning?"

"No, Momma," I said as I pointed to her. "Aren't YOU just a bundle of joy this morning?"

"No!" she said firmly.

"No?"

"No, no," she answered again.

"Well, what would make YOU full of joy this morning?"

Then I saw it. That familiar little mischievous grin spread slowly over her face, giving way to little giggles and a look in her eyes that said "joy" whether she could express it or not. A surprise came later when she was looking intently out the front door as she ate her breakfast. "What are you watching, Momma?"

She continued staring at Russell as he stood outside the fence getting mail out of the box.

"I was watching the preacher there," she answered as she ate another bite.

"What is he doing?" No response.

"Is he still there?" Not a word from her. "Is he coming back into the house?" No comment. She had said her piece and no amount of coaxing was going to get another word out of her. That sentence was the first in months; just hearing her voice at all had been a great blessing for me, but I yearned for more. The child was talking, almost as if learning words and phrases and I, the parent, was listening for every new syllable.

My journal entry written the very next day says it best.

Occasionally I catch just a tiny glimpse, then, sure enough there she is. That glimpse into her very soul; that sparkle, that knowing. All of Momma is there; hidden deep inside. Sometimes I look into Momma's eyes and I see the real Mom; the one that cared for me, that listened to me, that loved me. How I miss her.

It hurt so much when her familiar expressions were not followed by some conversation. In order for me to be able to hear her sweet voice at all, I often coaxed her into reading a page for me from her little books. Hearing just one sentence was enough to keep me going a little longer; enough to remind me that sweet little lady really was Mother.

After dressing her one morning she looked up into my face. I quickly kissed her and smiled. "Gotta catch those smoochies when you can, Momma. We need those hugs and kisses." She smiled and repeated, "Need those hugs and kisses." A few minutes later as she was resting in her chair, I heard sounds. "I…ah… Ah I…we…ah…I ah…"

I rubbed her back while watching her face. She was looking around and clearly struggling to get some words out. My heart ached for her. When it became clear to me the words would not come, then I moved in front of her, asked her about breakfast and got her giggling about which one of us would be going to "cook" the Wheaties. "Oh, Lord, how I love her. Such a child she is right now. Protect her. Help me."

I wrote the following in my journal after watching her eat one day:

Your spoon comes methodically to your mouth and you take one bite after another. Your hand is so steady as not to spill a drop. I watch for some time as you gingerly continue to eat your cereal. But, there is nothing in the bowl; it is empty. Oh, Momma, how I miss you. Where have you gone?

As I reflect on the many hours you and I have spent through the years sharing about the beauty of God's creation, I miss you even more. We now live in the midst of beautiful woods which provide great views from any direction. Your eyes brighten as I tell you of the deer feeding outside the kitchen window, the turkey under the walnut trees, or the latest escapades of the resident groundhog or the squirrel family. As I elaborate on every new adventure, Mother, you have all the wonder of a small child on your face. Then, so like a child, you settle back into your own little world. How I yearn for a good, long visit like we had in days gone by or a long stroll together through the woods. I can sit on our new deck with my eyes closed and picture you sitting next to me with our glasses of tea, but it is not to be.

There are many conversations I wish I would have had with my mother. Things we should have and could have talked about but didn't. Fear of approaching touchy subjects kept us from talking about some things. Yet I am sure making or taking time to visit was the biggest factor. How very, very important it is to learn all we can from our senior citizens while they are able to share. Mother had stories, past and present, locked up forever in her mind that only she and God knew.

Even without the benefit of verbal conversation, there were some moments too priceless for words. I recall walking past Mother's chair to go to the kitchen one day. I stopped to lean down and kiss her forehead. She looked up at me with glistening eyes and a tiny smile. As I touched her, she held my hand and gently squeezed. She held on tightly as I turned to leave. I didn't go. Nothing, not one thing in the entire world was more important than this moment. We cuddled and nuzzled with our hands joined, and I kissed her forehead again and again. She moved my hand to her lips a time or two and I felt a gentle kiss. What a blessed, blessed time with my Mom! Oh, what I could have so easily missed had I just patted her and went on to work. "God, You ordain my time so that I can love and care for those You've entrusted to me. Thank You for Your child, my Momma!"

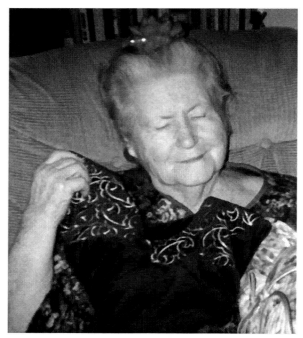

New Christmas Robe
"Is I pretty?"

FACING LIFE'S REALITIES

↩

*I*t was about 3:00 in the morning, and I could see Mother was not in her bed. I saw her lying on the floor in a lifeless huddle of covers and body. My heart pounded as I wondered what had happened, and if she was going to be okay. She heard me enter her room, and stared up at me with a puzzled look on her face.

"Whatcha doing there, Momma?"

"I's just here."

"How come you are on the floor? Did you just get tired of that old bed?"

"I did. I just got tired of that old bed."

She smiled so sweetly and winked at me as if to say, "Everything is okay down here." By giving her gentle love pats all over, I determined that she had not hurt or broken anything on her way to the floor.

"Well, Momma, would you like to just sleep there where you are? We could just have a slumber party right here."

Giggle, giggle.

"Think it's an okay idea, huh?"

"I do."

With her approval I prepared her for her slumber party. It was thankfully a warm night and the carpet felt comfortable. I snuggled her up in blankets and fluffed a pillow for her head. Before I got the light turned off, she was fast asleep. And I was thanking God for protecting her again.

This was the beginning of a whole new world of changes for her and for me as well. The first two years Mom was with us she had been pretty spry and moved about freely. She would go to bed when it was time with very little assistance and she would stay there all night. Even so, I got up and down throughout the night to make sure she was comfortable and sleeping well.

Several times now I had found her sitting on the edge of the bed, generally asleep and slumped over a bit. Waking her up gently, I would help her back into the bed, and she would usually make it through the rest of the night. This meant that I would sleep in the living room, just outside her door, so I could check on her more often.

It was becoming more apparent to Russell and I that we would have to get a hospital bed for her safety. Excitement grew as I explained the benefits of her new bed. I felt it was important to always advise her concerning any changes, and even ask her permission as we did this time. She seemed happier when she felt she had a part in whatever changes we made that would have an effect on her. There were lots of benefits; the smaller bed would give her more room to move around, and we would be able to raise and lower her head for comfort. Yes, excitement mounted as we prepared for this brand new bed.

The bed arrived and she watched eagerly as I made it up with fresh linens and a new pillow just for her. We both looked forward to bedtime to try it out.

The excitement didn't last long before reality hit. Getting her into the bed had been a snap and she looked very happy. I had taken the safety bar completely off the front so it wouldn't hurt her short chunky legs as she sat on the edge of the bed. Now, as I lifted the bar and brought it toward the bed, she looked frightened and helpless.

"Momma, this is your helper bar; you will like it."

She didn't look like she was going to like it at all. Part of that may have been a reflection of my expressions as I thought of putting up the safety bar. This was going to lock her in for the night like a baby in a crib. We both realized that this was another part of taking away her freedom. Now she would have to wait for me to get her out of bed, because she would not understand how to let the bar down on her own. Getting a bell for her to ring when she needed help would not have worked for her either.

I felt like I was locking my mother in a jail cell; it was the most horrible feeling yet. But, for safety's sake, I put the bar on and pulled her covers up under her chin. After giving her lots of hugs and reassuring words about how much this bar would aide her, I left her and turned out the light.

Earlier that evening, I had watched her doze in her big green chair with her feet propped on a pillow. Her hands were in her lap on a saucer where a sandwich had been. Still firmly held between her thumbs and forefingers was a single piece of crust; held securely by both hands as she slept. Her hair was pulled back revealing age lines seldom seen when she was awake and full of smiles. And she looked old, tired, frail, and so helpless and dependent; childlike. Back in the living room, I cried and cried and cried. "God, help Mother and me to adjust to this new time in our journey. Remind me often that this is a necessary process, even though my heart hurts so."

One of the most difficult decisions for me was putting Mother into diapers. I knew we had to do something because the leaks and accidents were becoming more frequent as she lost control of bodily functions. I was aware of Depends and other adult garments for this purpose, but she was my mother and this would not be an easy adjustment for either of us.

I couldn't call them diapers. When we tried the first pair, I told Mom I was going to get her some new britches that would fit her better. I explained that it would help her stay dry and help me to keep things cleaner. She seemed to accept that idea at the time.

As I put the first pair on her, I said we would need to try these new britches for awhile and see how they work. She nodded in agreement but I could see that she wasn't really happy about them. One time she said "These aren't britches!"

"Well, no," I replied. "But I think they will work, don't you think so?" She smiled and we continued.

I changed my mother's diapers like a child for five years and was grateful for them. I did not, however, ever call them "diapers".

Mother had many, many, many accidents. Like a baby she had to be cleaned up often and so did the floor. And, yes, sometimes I wanted her to wait to go to the bathroom; just hold it until we got on the potty. I didn't always feel too energetic myself, and I was not anxious to change her and clean up the mess.

When I was a child, I am sure my mother cleaned me up again and again. Our family lived in the backwoods and she had to go down the hill to get buckets of water, scrub and scrub those cloth diapers, and hang them to dry. All of this in the same room where we all ate, slept and lived. We had kerosene lamps, a wood stove, and a path out back to the outhouse. My brother was two years younger than me, so she had two of us to care for while Dad was at work. She would tell me of times when she left us on the top of the hill with our dog as a babysitter while she scurried down to get some water hoping we would not toddle off into the woods. With no electricity or neighbors nearby, she was pretty much on her own. Surely she was often tired, weary, and impatient.

God says in Philippians 4:8 TLB,

. . . Fix your thoughts on what is true and good and right. Think about things that are pure and lovely, and dwell on the fine, good things in others. Think about all you can praise God for and be glad about it.

God's Word called me to remember Mother's pure love for me and our family, and her love for life's simple things. I was once again reminded of how blessed I was to have the awesome privilege to care for her. I was so thankful for running water, clean towels and washcloths, my washer and dryer, plenty of soaps and deodorizers, room enough to do my work, and disposable diapers.

Mother's emotional well being was far more important than a little mess here and there. When she first started dribbling on the way to the bathroom, I used large area rugs and matching runners to cover areas where she would be walking. Vinyl under each rug kept the floor protected and stitching those all together kept her from tripping on the edges. She actually enjoyed her new "runway" and took great pride in following it to her room or to the bathroom. More vinyl covered her chair cushions and washable fabric throws over them kept her skin clean and comfortable.

Our house always smelled fresh and clean thanks to a large variety of cleaning products and a small, well-used electric shampooer.

When little children have accidents they are quickly forgiven because we understand that they cannot help it. I knew that Mother would never, ever make such messes on purpose if the choice was hers. A visitor in our home commented once on how well we handled such things. I quickly responded that this was no different than what they faced each day with their small children.

"Yes, we do have little ones to care for," was the compassionate reply, "but our children will grow up and your 'child' never will."

"Perhaps not, but she will be a happy child, and well cared for as long as she is here."

Caring for someone, really caring, is so much more than providing basic needs. It is being sensitive to their changing desires and physical abilities, and then adjusting accordingly. When I first began to realize she was becoming unsteady and in danger of falling, I gave her a three-legged cane. She clearly did not think she needed it, but did slowly begin to use it. When the physical therapist presented her with a walker, Mother said it would be "good to have if I ever need it." That was Momma!

Momma slowed a lot through the years and often rested many times on the way to her room. Three times every day I would encourage each step she took. "Come on, Momma, you can make it. One more step with this foot. Move your leg, Momma. Just a little. That's it. Great! Now the other one."

No amount of encouragement would work. If I put a chair under her and let her rest a bit, she could make a few more steps, if she chose. Sometimes she chose to stand there with no signs of moving any time soon. When I grew weary of smiling or of trying to understand how to help her, it seemed God was always there with just what I needed to continue on. Clear as a picture I could hear all those same words coming to me from my Mother. She encouraged me when I learned to walk, to ride a bike, to drive, to recover after an illness. Suddenly I wasn't so tired anymore. "Come on, Momma, you can do it. I will help you!"

It soon became difficult for her to walk very far without tiring. That meant the wheelchair arrived next. She got used to it pretty quickly. Perhaps she realized she was just getting too tired to do much else. It was a challenge for me at first; pushing someone in a wheelchair looks so simple. It isn't! Mother's size and short stature worked against her in the wheelchair. I almost dumped her before I learned how to navigate well. Because she could not always reason things out, I also had to remind her to sit back in the chair before I moved her.

I have a new appreciation for people confined to wheelchairs and those who must transport them. You have to learn to maneuver this awkward chair in all sorts of environments. "Handicap Accessible" does not necessarily mean it's easy. Getting to your destination from the handicap entrance may mean a long walk through a busy clinic or hospital. Mother always looked frailer in the wheelchair. We had to stoop down to her level to communicate. The edge of the seat often hurt the back of her short legs. Her feet did not touch the floor. The wheelchair may have been easier and faster for us to use, but it was not better for her. We only used the chair when she was really sick, or to get her outside and into a transport van. I always encouraged her to walk as much as possible, even if she had to rest several times along the way. I thought it would help her circulation and her energy level if she could keep those muscles active.

When Mother's recliner wore out and I went shopping for a replacement, I considered a lift chair. It was becoming increasingly difficult for her to get out of her chair, even with help. She didn't seem to have the strength or understanding to simply stand up and reach her walker.

There are so many factors to consider in a mechanical chair. On many of the less-expensive models, the back reclines as the foot rest rises. This would mean that someone had to practically be lying down in order to have their feet elevated. I did not want Mother lying down all the time. It was important that she sit up and keep those back muscles strong. I knew if she got completely helpless, I could not care for her at home.

I looked at several of the more expensive models and even brought one home for Mother to try. My short, stubby mother was lost in that chair. Not only did the chair not fit her, I began to realize that leaving her in an unattended motorized chair was an invitation to disaster.

About the time I got her settled in a new, small recliner, Mother began to lose weight. This meant adding pillows behind her as well as under her legs to protect them from the rigid edge of the recliner's foot-rest. Extra pillows also meant extra pads to keep them dry. I used heavy cloth ones at first, then started using the disposable ones when possible. It was a matter of weighing the cost of running the washer constantly against the cost of the disposable pads. We used a pillow on her lap for a table since a tray by itself would slide right off her lap. Perhaps you get the idea; caregiving is a constant adjustment of one thing or another. Circumstances change from day to day and caregivers must be ready to change with them. The primary goal is simply to make life easier for our loved one.

Food was another learning experience in this second childhood of Mother's. I was determined to the last that she would always feed herself if at all possible. I knew that if I started feeding her, I would always have to do it, and she would lose that last thread of independence. We sure had some messes! I just bought bigger bibs, towels and throw rugs and allowed her plenty of time to enjoy her food.

Once I watched Momma as she seemed to be stringing chicken onto her fork. She clearly had done this for some time as there were tiny slivers of chicken breast on her, the table, the floor, etc.

"Hi, Momma! Whatcha doin'?"

Silence, then a smile and . . ."I was. . . . I was a makin' flowers!"

"Great, looks like you're doin' a good job."

"I is."

"You know what I thought you were makin'?"

"No."

"I thought you were makin a mess!"

There were giggles and giggles, and the expression of a little girl having a good time. I took her plate and cleaned the mess as she watched, still grinning at me.

"Do you need something else to eat or are you full?"

"I is full."

I would have to give her a sandwich later because, in true child-like fashion, she wore much more of her lunch than she ate.

And what a child she had become. It took so little to please her. She was quite content with a hamburger and a colorful cartoon to watch. Old sit-coms or westerns on television or a Gaither Gospel Music show would keep her occupied for hours.

I don't know when the baby talk began. It seemed that, as she began behaving more like a child, she talked more like one. And I noticed myself using baby talk with her, especially when kidding her about something she had done. I think phrases such as, "You is a treasure, Mommy," were short and full of warm fuzzies for both of us. For several years, she just wouldn't pay attention to long conversations or complex sentences.

As time passed, Russell and I had to be more careful about leaving her by herself to eat as she would stuff her mouth full like a chipmunk. When I realized that she had half a hamburger in her mouth, I had to use my finger to dig it all out. Well, here was just one more change to keep us on the alert.

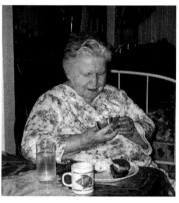 Sometimes Mother would slowly pour her drink into her plate filled with food and then play in it. So like a child. I think memory loss can be a blessing. My neat, tidy mother would not at all be pleased with herself if she really understood her plight.

I had not expected the childlike behavior changes. It is true that she was usually happy and seemed content no matter what was happening. However, she would also pout like a small child when she felt left out. If I brought Russell something to eat, anything at all, she seemed to think she needed something even if she had just eaten a large meal. If I didn't give her something, she would scoot forward in her chair and stare at him with a frown on her face. She evidently didn't understand why she had been left out.

When our children visited, they would often

bring her a candy bar. It was unmistakably hers and hers alone. Asking her to share usually brought a kind look and a smile, but no bite of her bar. When given bags of candy or boxes of chocolate at Christmas, I would have to move them when she wasn't looking or she would eat an entire box or bag of candy in one sitting.

Feeding little children takes time; so did feeding Momma. I recall wanting to leave for a meeting in Springfield and going in to get Mother's plate before we left. She should have already finished her breakfast and been ready to move into her recliner. As I watched her eat, I could tell that "ready" was not going to happen anytime soon. I watched as she carefully put the spoon into her bowl, lifted one single bran flake and slowly put it into her mouth meticulously chewing it up. Then she took a small swallow of juice, sat the glass back down, and picked up the spoon to get about ¼ teaspoon of milk in it. That was followed by a sip of juice, a tiny flake of cereal, another bit of milk on the spoon. This process was repeated over and over again. "Lord, she seems to really be enjoying her meal today, and I think I am getting an ulcer!"

Was it God who nudged me to remind me of my priorities? After all, look at the great exercise her arm was getting. Did God send that pleasant aroma of happiness into her room? Life outside the house would have to wait because my mother was enjoying her meal.

Another journal entry describes one of the
many new habits Mother acquired:

> *Clack, clack, clack; clackety, clack! She's gently tap-*
> *ping her glass on her teeth. A few weeks ago she*
> *would do this occasionally for a little bit. Now it's*
> *quite frequent. She stops if we look at her and be-*
> *gins again when we turn away. When I ask her*
> *what she is doing, she immediately quits tapping*
> *and stares at me. I'm not sure what it means, is it*
> *just a nervous reaction? Does she want something,*
> *perhaps attention? Her glass usually has some-*
> *thing in it. Maybe she somehow gets some comfort*
> *from hearing the rhythm.*

One night after letting her tap, tap for about
ten minutes, I gathered the dishes and reached for her
glass. She nodded when asked if she was finished and
she gave the glass to me. Then she stared at the glass
and at me as if asking why I took it away from her. She
sadly watched me until I was out of sight. I knew I had
to buy some plastic glasses and cups so that she could
enjoy them without the threat of broken glass. It would
also keep me from feeling like a criminal for taking her
enjoyment away.

Some habits were more difficult to deal with.
"Spit-choo! Plop!"

"Momma, what are you doing?"

No response. A few minutes later, "Spit-choo!
Plop!"

"Momma, you cannot spit on the floor." Blank

stare. I sensed a definite "I can if I want to" expression. My tidy little momma was purposefully spitting on the floor! Efforts to stop her were to no avail. The only answer seemed to be to keep antibacterial cleaners and cleaning cloths handy.

Thankfully, like many of her other habits, this would soon give way to something else, but it wore on her caregiver. I wanted to yell at her, "You know better than that! Behave yourself! You are making work for me!" I wanted to paddle her bottom; I wanted to cry. I could only love her through it and pray as I assured her once again, "Mommy, you is a mess, but I loves you anyway!"

A friend once asked me what her doctor said about her habits like clacking the glass on her teeth and spitting. I never did tell him about it. Another person asked why Mother quit talking; what caused it? I don't know. I didn't tell her doctor that either. It's not that I meant to keep these things from him. So many seemingly more serious things surfaced with her care each week and they became the priority. The clacking and spitting, like many of her other habits, were temporary. As far as the loss of speech, that was a gradual thing. After her first stay in the hospital, she never talked much. I wasn't sure if she couldn't speak, or just simply didn't think it necessary. Early on, with coaxing, she would say a few sentences when she was in the mood.

Hindsight is always 20/20. Now I have cause to wonder if, with earlier detection, we could have preserved her speaking ability a little longer. I don't know. I do know that in life we make many decisions based on what we know at the time, and then we live with the consequences. For me, I find great peace in knowing that, after much prayer, our family did the best we could for Mother each and every day she was entrusted to us.

There is one thing a caregiver learns right away: nothing, absolutely nothing, stays the same. We gave Mother the television remote so she could choose what she wanted to watch on television. At the time, she was still able to move from room to room. Late one night we were awakened by very, very loud music. Mother was in her chair just pushing buttons. Did she wake up thinking it was day, or could she just not sleep?

Soon after the episode with the television, we moved the remote from her table. It was clear that she could no longer understand all those buttons. As time went on, we gradually removed other things: straws, Kleenex, napkins, any chewable items. Bit by bit her environment was becoming a safe place for a child.

It was the child that appeared most often in sickness. Once, when Mother was lying on her bed struggling with a nose and chest full of congestion and sneezing constantly, I gave her a tissue to clear her sinuses out, but she didn't understand what to do with it. She took the tissue, neatly folded it and held it in her hand, still sniffing and sneezing and dribbling.

"Momma, blow your nose," I told her as I guided her tissue to her nose. Her eyes lit up as she understood and she blew and blew and cleared her nose out pretty well.

"Now cough." Blank stare. "Momma, can you cough real hard for me?"

"No."

"Try."

No response, just a smile. Meanwhile she kept sneezing a little.

"Momma, you sound like a train. Choo, choo! Choo, choo!"

She got so tickled at my silliness that she automatically coughed and cleared that congestion right out of her throat. Mission accomplished!

When she had a bladder or vaginal infection, caring for her private parts was extremely difficult. The child did not understand. "Isn't this yucky, Mom?" I asked as I applied the medicine according to the directions on the package.

"Yes," she replied with a little frown.

"I don't like this, do you?"

"No!" It was quite clear that she would just as soon I quit applying the medicines and leave her alone.

"Well, the doctor said this is very, very important in order to help you get well quicker. Let's just pray that you get well really quick, okay?"

"Okay," she answered with a relaxed look of approval on her face. A few simple words of comfort and an explanation of what I was doing had eased her mind and helped us over another hurdle.

Sometimes when Momma would have a real bad sick spell, she would pull my hand to her mouth and chew on my knuckle much like a baby does. She would hold tightly if I tried to pull away. "Oh, little girl, I wonder if you are, in some small way, getting the nurturing you missed as a child. My mother, my child, I want to tenderly care for you every minute of every day that you are with us."

I spent many hours holding her hand while watching her sleep. How I hungered to have her awaken as the real Mom; the one I could confide in and visit with, laugh and cry, recollect old times and plan new ones. I miss her so much while she is still here; how will I ever make it when she is gone?

HIRED STRANGERS
OR CONCERNED CAREGIVERS

ᥣ

"The home health agency is going to send someone out to help care for Mother several days a week. I'm not really sure I am ready to have strange people in and out of our home all the time."

Russell was quick to reply. "You can handle it. After all, we have always welcomed anyone into our home without notice."

"But, I don't know what to expect when they come or what to have them do for me. I really prefer to just do things myself." Being in the ministry, we *were* used to having people in our home often, but this would be totally different. Now I had to trust strangers to care for my mother and to clean my house or do my laundry. Mary and Jessie had become like family by now, but I knew they could not do it all.

Mother had reached the point where she could not do very much on her own. I knew in my heart extra help was necessary for her and for me as well. When home health and respite care became available to her, I was both relieved and nervous. It was, at first, a challenge for me to not "help" the helpers. I had been so protective of her and responsible for her total care.

Realizing those caring for her would not really know any of us, I made small information cards and tacked several in each room. Russell and I had some cards with us at all times, and kept copies in both vehicles. Since Mother could not communicate her needs, we had to have some assurance that those caring for her in an emergency would have the information they required to care for her properly.

The colorful cards listed the medicines and dosages she was currently taking; any allergies, her legal name and what to call her, her date of birth, the physical address of our home, her physician and hospital and the phone numbers for each, her insurance companies and their phone numbers and addresses, the phone number of the transportation van, and the number for our preferred mortuary. It stated on the card that she was living with her daughter and son-in-law and listed our names, cell phone number, the cars we drove and the license numbers of each. I knew this was necessary should anyone need to locate us in an emergency. I stated the caregiver should not hesitate to call 911 anytime there was a question concerning her well being.

I did not know what to expect when the time came for the agency to send out a caregiver. When she arrived, it was apparent that we were both nervous. It turns out that was to be the first day for both of us; Mother was her first client and she was our first caregiver. I knew when I saw her sincere smile, and heard her name that God had sent Enid Rauh to us. *Enid,* Oklahoma had been a special place to Mother in her young adult years.

Enid was a gifted caregiver. From the first time she entered our home, Mother was her first priority. She stopped by Mother's chair and introduced herself before ever talking with me. She fluffed Mother's pillow, made her comfortable, and then joined me in the kitchen for details of the job. Enid was going to be in our home three or four times every week. My main requirement for any caregiver was simply to make sure Mom was comfortable and happy, and to sit with her while Mother ate her meals.

Any possible concerns quickly vanished as I watched the two of them over the weeks and years that followed. There was real love between Enid and Mom; Mother's eyes would light up when she saw Enid step up onto the porch. From pampering her to playing the piano and singing for her, Enid spoiled her and that pleased me immensely. She treated Mother with respect and dignity, as an adult with specific needs and tender feelings. She was always joyful whether cleaning up a potty mess or patiently helping Mother finish a meal. We would often come home to a meal in the crock pot for our entire family; what a pleasant surprise to open the door to the aroma of a home cooked meal prepared by someone else's hands!

I know that many agencies caution their workers not to get personally involved with their clients; that they are there to do a job. I know too, that not all women have the personality or talents to do everything that Enid did. I do think however, that those who accept the responsibility to work for someone in any capacity should really show respect for those in their care. We quickly learned to recognize those who were simply working for a paycheck as opposed to those who genuinely cared for Mother.

We usually had a bath aide and perhaps respite care or a housekeeper three times a week. However, at one point we had at least two different people each day of the week: nurse, bath aide, housekeeper, physical therapist, occupational therapist, and speech therapist. All of this activity was sometimes overwhelming.

Coordinating our schedules was difficult at first. Russell and I tried to plan our meals, appointments, and other trips around these women and their schedules. I was determined to be home when a worker was scheduled to come so I would know who was there and what they did. The truth soon became evident; if I had to be home anyway, I might as well be doing the work.

Russell and I had to make some tough choices for the best of all concerned. We did much praying and based each decision on what we felt God would have us do. For some, that may seem a little unrealistic or simplistic. To us, it came down to one question: do we put our trust in people or in God? We were certain that God had provided this particular home in this city for us, and He knew better than we what our needs would be. We had to trust Him to care for Mother. We decided that we did not always need to be home when a bath aide or other home health worker was scheduled to come. Because we live in a very small, farming community, we also chose to leave the doors unlocked, allowing people the freedom to come and go as they had need.

I feel I must note here that I am aware leaving the door unlocked would not work for everyone. These are very personal, extremely tough decisions that must be made on an individual basis. For us, this was the most natural avenue. Mother, Russell and I had all grown up in homes with unlocked doors in small communities and were thankful to be in a rural community now. We had been accustomed to people from church dropping by when they were in the neighborhood and actually relied upon them continuing that practice. For me, personally, I felt more secure knowing people could get in, should there be an emergency, than I would have with Mother behind a locked door. I should also note that we were not ever gone all day without knowing for sure there was someone that we knew we could trust with Mother.

Many of the caregivers were great at what they did, but some caused me to doubt the wisdom of having any outside help. Agencies have even said to me that they did the best they could to get capable workers, but there simply was not enough experienced help available. Sometimes a new girl would not show up when scheduled, and not bother to call to let us know. I once returned home to find Mother exactly where we had left her, with no lunch and no care. This limited our going far unless we were very sure someone would be with her.

As I realized that workers changed frequently, I thought it was time for more notes. I prepared a little notebook of simple things such as the snacks Mother enjoyed, how to cut up her food, and what her daily routine was. It was necessary they give her a spoon instead of a sharp fork. They were told to allow her to nibble on her food all afternoon if she wanted. There were instructions on how to put her plate on a pillow on her lap. I suggested they always talk with her about each thing they did.

Much of what I wrote down was common sense things that a person in the home every day would automatically do. But, for instance, an aide coming only one day a week might not consider closing the blinds before she left at night so that Mother would not be fearful of the darkened window.

Another list was made telling where things are kept: cleaning supplies, extra paper goods, coffee makings, gowns, shoes, linens, extra skin crèmes, etc. This list not only helped the new girls as they came, it also helped me keep at least a little order around the house.

In the notebook I wrote:

Mother's entire world revolves around what happens inside this home. You need to know that she loves attention, hugs, laughing, to be included, eating almost anything, listening to you talk, and music. She is more at ease when you treat her like a normal adult and expect a reaction from her when you ask something.

One day I was startled to come home from the store and hear loud voices coming from Mother's room. I rushed in to see what was happening. Mother was on her commode looking forlorn as two women were giving her a bath. Apparently, one was teaching the other; though it was hard to tell who was doing the training. One was scrubbing her back hard while the other scrubbed her legs. They were talking loudly, not to Mom, but to each other. I watched for a few minutes as they continued without letting them know that I was in there. As my frustration grew, I chose carefully how to deal with the situation. It seemed that my first words should be addressed to my helpless little Mother.

"Mommy, you sure are getting a lot of attention today. Does that bath feel good?" She smiled and looked at the two of them with concern.

"Maybe they could just be a little easier on you. Would that be a good thing?"

"It would be a good thing," she answered.

I stopped them and asked could they please

handle her gently and talk to her, not to each other. I asked them to think about the fact that she was a very old lady with tender skin who sat around all day long. She did not need to be scrubbed hard to get clean.

All too often, I had to remind caregivers that they were there to care for Mom, and their attention should be directed to her. She was a special lady, and she needed to be treated as such at all times. At the very least, they could smile at her once in awhile or pat her hand as they went by. Conversation needed to be addressed to her, whether or not she would respond.

It was impossible to depend on what I was told about the events of her day. I listened to one glowing account of how well Mother had eaten her lunch, yet later I found most of her food in the trash can. It was time consuming to help her eat; sometimes it meant feeding her most of the meal, but it was necessary. My preference was for the girls to encourage her to eat on her own, but many would not give her the time she needed.

I also asked that the television be left on a gospel music station or cartoons or old stories like *Little House on the Prairie*. Mother enjoyed those programs and was more content when she had something to watch. I was concerned that her brain be cared for, too. I did not think she needed anything to listen to that would cause her to worry or become anxious. Was I being overly protective? Could she really handle more mentally than I gave her credit for? If I erred, it was going to be on the side of a happy, content older lady who deserved to be spoiled.

Too many times I would find the caregiver sitting in a chair watching a soap opera with volume blaring while Mother sat needing to be changed and cleaned up. If the television or the radio was on the right channel, the volume often would be so low that Mother couldn't hear it. This happened all too often with Christian radio stations in particular and I wondered if the aide just didn't want to hear it herself. I was not trying to convert anyone else. My Mother needed the familiar happy sounds. She would sit up and listen to music for long periods of time often tapping her fingers and toes to the rhythm.

One big help for me was the home health nurse who came once a month or more as needed. I had always felt anxious about making decisions concerning Mother's health, and it was great to have someone who really understood her needs and could explain different options to me.

Another great help was the various first responders or on-call emergency personnel. In our rural area of Missouri, 911 emergency calls were frequently answered by well-trained, often unpaid volunteers. I was so thankful for those who gave so selflessly to help the rest of us. Reality is, in this quiet family community, those who answered our calls were probably happy for a chance to use their skills.

One day while Mother was walking toward the bathroom with her walker, her knees just seemed to go limp. She quickly slipped down onto the floor in that crowded hallway still holding onto her walker. "Now we are in a big mess! How are we ever going to get Mother up from this floor? Here in this tiny space, halfway through the bathroom doorway, is the worse place she could be. There is absolutely no room for us to even get around her to try to lift her." This time I could see no way out of our predicament.

"Relax, I'll just call 911," my wise husband quickly replied.

The expertise and patience of those who responded still overwhelms me. They were so kind and gentle with my mother and kept her at ease in a difficult situation. With proper equipment and savvy, Mother was back in her chair in no time.

Therapists too, are indispensable. Therapy takes on a whole new meaning when you see it in action. I was continually amazed at how just a few simple exercises could get Mother up and moving. Goals would be set for her and she would try her best to meet them. The patience and perseverance of some have put therapists high on my list of admired professions. Time and again when I was so sure Mother could not or would not stand or walk again, I would be thrilled to experience the joy of watching her take tiny strides toward wholeness once more.

Susan Richardson was clearly Mother's favorite physical therapist. Susan just seemed to be able to motivate her when no one else could. "You can do this," she would say. "Just try a little harder to stand up." Patiently Susan watched and waited. "You can. You really can. I have faith in you. Let's show Susie how it's done." Once again Mother would pull herself up, grab hold of the walker, and off she would go (slowly).

I originally wondered why any occupational therapist would be called for someone who had no occupation (my healthcare knowledge was obviously very impaired). I soon learned they were there to help Mother with everyday essentials such as combing her hair, washing her face and doing light chores about the house. These things helped her continue to be at least somewhat independent. Along with helping Mother relearn these simple tasks, the therapists also helped me to recognize ways I could keep Mother occupied.

By the time I figured out why we needed occupational therapy, a speech therapist was sent out to evaluate Mother and my learning continued. Speech therapy was a great aid with her communication skills; even when words were gone. It is amazing how many ways other than through speech we can communicate our needs and wants.

The mere fact that Mother had all these nice people giving her personal care inspired her to do her best. This was apparent right away when our Mary first came to help us. When any aide arrived, Mother would readily perk up and be ready for the attention that would be focused on her and her alone.

In preparing to write this book, I asked a few of our best healthcare workers what they would tell an individual who was hired to care for someone in their home. Here are some of their suggestions:

1. Remember you are invading the privacy of that family. Respect their home.

2. Don't bring your troubles into that home. They need you to be happy so don't add to their load.

3. Care for that person as you would want someone to care for your parent or child.

4. Remember, no matter how difficult the client, she is still a person, not an object.

5. Learn the technical aspects of care and then adjust to the person.

6. Help them to not feel ashamed when they have accidents or have difficulty remembering things.

7. Be extremely patient with their progress or lack of it.

8. Realize they may be expressing truth as they understand it to the best of their ability.

9. Find out the name your client uses, and use it. The client will respond better to names they are familiar with.

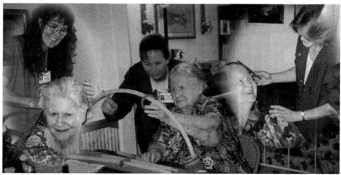

Enid   Ginger   Mary

UPS & DOWNS OF CAREGIVING

⌒

"How's your Mother? Is she doing well today?"
"She's doing great today. Thanks for asking."
In reality this was not a question I could answer with
any certainty. One day she would be unable to sit up
and the next day she might be walking with her walker.
My hopes would rise as we would go through several
weeks of progress only to fall again when she would
take a turn for the worse.

A few of my journal entries best describe the
ups and downs of caring. The first was written in January
five years before Mother died:

> *Mother is watching the parade of colorful birds
> feeding at the feeders hung outside the window,
> including more than a dozen bright red cardinals. The sun is coming up over the hill adding
> diamonds to the snow-packed yard. Crystal limbs
> hang heavy and beautiful in the shimmering sun-*

light. After days of being extremely ill, she is doing great and going to be okay. The promise of a new day beckons and I am ready! It's a new year, a time for renewed commitments; hopes for a better tomorrow.

Only three days later I wrote:

I have such an overwhelming sense of my need for the Lord today. Mom's been so sick again. I wonder if she'll need to be hospitalized. I checked on her then sat down with my Bible. Before turning a page, I felt these tears run down my cheek and my spirit praying, 'Lord, I need You. I am so totally helpless. I cannot make these decisions concerning Mother and our family without You. Little seemingly ordinary decisions loom heavy in my heart and I need You so much.'

One week later the journal continues:

I'm so excited I can barely contain myself. Earlier as I snuggled on Russell's shoulder and we talked, I felt a renewed sense of wonder and peace. When I took Mother's second cup of coffee to her room, she was as bright-eyed and full of smiles as she ever had been. She had brushed her own hair and was eager to face this new day. And so am I.

Time passes and again I write:

Momma's weakened so much these past few weeks. She is non-responsive as I try to talk to her. She is very slow to get up from the chair and she has to rest every two steps. Is it time to use the wheelchair or will that only allow her to become more feeble? When will I know? How can I tell for sure? I want what's best for her well being. Am I helping her by pushing her more or am I contributing to the problem by wearing her out? Help!

Again a page from my journal dated January 20, 2003, proves helpful to describe the feelings and trauma of caregiving:

A Hoyer Lift! Now the nurse is telling us that Mother may have to be left in bed more often unless we choose to get a Hoyer Lift to help move her in and out of bed. It's getting so confusing to me; I do not understand why others cannot care for her as I do. I pray for guidance and patience and understanding. I do not want to be hard to get along with, but I don't want to be walked on either. The nurse and social worker had explained to me that aides reported that they could simply not handle my mother without this help.

After they finished asking me pages of questions concerning Mother and her care and her abilities, the nurse requested I get her up from her chair. Mother smiled so pretty for them and stood with very little help (better than she had done all week). Then she walked a few steps. I could hear them mumbling, 'My, oh my, look at her go!' Looking at me the nurse asked, 'What is their problem! She is not difficult to move.' I wanted to hug them both.

I thanked God in my heart for His care. Finally someone was with me and for me. We concluded that those caring for her need to give her more time to do things and not rush her. They need to let her do as much as possible on her own even if it means allowing her to set her own pace. In my heart I know that she will continue to lose strength and the will to do more. I am ready to accept the fact that additional equipment and helps will be necessary sometime. But not now!

A few months later, Susan would have her walking all the way to the fireplace with only one stop. Her muscles had strengthened and she could get in and out of bed with minimal help. Then in a few short days, she was weak and feeble again with a temperature of 103. Over and over again hopes would rise and then suddenly fall as her condition changed. Whatever the circumstances, we continued to do our best to make her happy and comfortable, and to shower her with hugs and kisses, all the while encouraging her to do as much as possible on her own.

One great tool that proved to be very handy was a gait belt. The gait belt was a very wide, long belt with a buckle that fastened much like a safety belt in a car. A therapist had taught us how to position it properly around Mother's body and how to use it to help her sit or walk safely. Although skeptical at first, I became thankful for such a simple but valuable tool.

Over time I learned the necessity of keeping good records of her medications and her reactions to them. Tracking her medications helped us here at home as well as the doctors when changes were necessary. Over the years, we must have filled out a mountain of paperwork concerning Mother's health. Even with my background as a secretary, the endless records and forms seemed overwhelming at times. There was so much that I really didn't understand. What do people do who cannot read well or comprehend all the paperwork?

During eight years of caring for Mother we were in and out of hospitals and nursing homes more times than I care to number. A trip to see the doctor meant a long, bumpy ride in the hospital van and we put it off as long as possible. I always felt she was better at home than going through the ordeal of the rough trip and having strangers poke at her.

Often the changes in her condition came on unexpectedly. One morning after we had our usual giggles and silliness, I helped her stand and prepared her to sit on her commode. Russell had waited as he always did for the okay from me before he left the house to run some errands. Since she had awakened so alert and happy, I told him to go on to town. I was sure we could manage without his help. About the time I heard him start the car, I noticed Momma's lips tighten and her face turn pale. Too late to stop him, I prayed that she would be okay. I quickly got her seated on the commode and I sat on the bed next to her. She was so white and frail-looking. Hugging her I could feel her anxious heart beat through her back. She was hurting and I could not fix it!

For an hour and a half all I could do is hold her and wipe her brow with a cool cloth. I knew I could not move her by myself. I sat on the edge of her bed the entire time, trying to comfort her. I had one arm around her shoulder and dared not lessen my grip for fear she would slip down onto the floor.

"You're doing much better now," I said with a smile. "It will be okay, Momma." She looked at me with half-opened eyes and a slim, trembling smile as if to say "I know it will." She needed to lie down and my arms were breaking, but when I moved her at all she seemed worse.

Was I ever thankful to hear Russell open the garage door! Even though she seemed to be rallying, we waited a short time before trying to stand her up. He held her while I rested. Our first attempt failed so we waited a little longer. When we got a good reaction including a little smile from her, we decided to try again. Over the years we had learned exactly how to hold her with one hand while moving furniture with the other. On this day, we positioned ourselves so that, once we stood her up, we could move the commode and slide her chair under her. Each of us had our specific task and it had to be done quickly.

This time, however, her legs were feeble and she was quickly slipping from our grip. Using our feet one of us moved the commode while the other moved her chair out of the way. Then while holding on to her with the gait belt, we carefully lowered her to the floor. I straightened her legs, pillowed her head, covered her with soft blankets, and patted her hand until she went to sleep.

About 2:00 p.m. she awoke bright eyed, smiling, and ready for some food. We had developed a good system for getting her up when she was able to help even a little. We both stood in front of her and each put one of her feet on one of ours. Then we simultaneously reached down and pulled her up with the gait belt while she held on to our free arms. It is difficult to try to describe this process to someone else, but it works beautifully. It is amazing how easy it was to get her up from the floor in this manner when she had even a little strength to stiffen her legs a bit.

Again I penned my feelings as I reflected on the day.

> *It gets so hard sometimes. I don't want to keep facing these issues and not knowing what to do. How can I tell where she hurts when she can't tell me? How do I know when to take her to the doctor or just try to treat the problem at home? If he can only give her another pill and send her back home, why go?*

I had always thought I would know when to put Mom into a nursing home. It would be when I could no longer physically care for her. Russell and I had discussed ways we could work together to give her good care as her needs changed. But her mental care was harder to deal with. It was not so cut and dried. Not so obvious to me, at least. I wondered sometimes if I was prolonging her life beyond her wishes. Would she want to be here in this condition if she really understood how limited her life was and how childlike she had become? I was but a child myself crying out to God for wisdom and comfort.

CAPTURE THE MOMENT

⌒

*B*eing Mother's full time caregiver was hard. It was difficult work, filled with day-to-day problems. Caring for Mom took all the energies and resources I had available and then some. It changed my priorities, it tied me down and wore me out; it was often a thankless job. Being Mother's caregiver was also a privilege, an awesome responsibility. The rewards each day were fabulous, when I took the time to look for them. It was an opportunity to encourage Mom every day of her life, a challenge to make her hurting soul feel happy and loved. The opportunity to give of myself in caring for Mom was truly a gift from God.

It was also a time for me to draw closer to God. I knew that I could never care for my mother on my own without His daily help. God answered the faithful prayers of others to give me strength, understanding and patience when I had nothing left to give.

I loved Momma so much that it hurt, but there were times when my personal feelings, desires, and yes, even needs, got in the way. Sometimes I found myself wanting to do something just for me instead of something for Russell or Mother. I wanted to walk away and not be encumbered by all that work and responsibility. As a full time caregiver, I simply had to find time to get away for my own well being. Many times I had insisted that others in the same situation take some time away from the ones for whom they cared. Until I was actually in that position, I could not understand how complicated a decision about taking time for myself could be.

At one point I just ached to go visit my brother and his wife Linda in Texas. Not only did I need the time away, Linda's cancer had returned and I wanted to spend some time with the two of them. Just as it seemed it might be possible, Mother had a two week period of being very, very sick. A cold turned into bronchitis and I feared pneumonia. An allergic reaction to medications resulted in a bad rash from head to toe. That and a temperature of 102 degrees prompted a trip to the emergency room. It was refreshing news to learn that it had not been pneumonia, and there were some new medicines that would take care of her problems. Back home her skin peeled off and she got a severe case of fungal infection, and her only bed sore in all those years. A few days later she was walking with her walker to the fireplace, with a little help, and managing better than she had in a long time. Me? I was finally on my way to Texas; yet it hurt so much to leave knowing I had left her care in someone else's hands.

How can I describe the peace of crawling into bed in Linda's guest room? I missed Mother dreadfully, even for these few days. But it was great to be able to go to bed without having to move her, change her, tuck her in bed, do some laundry, and plan the next day's menu, etc. I prayed often for God to grant me a long time to continue caring for her; it was an honor and a privilege. I also thanked Him for those much-needed times of refreshing.

Caring for Mother would have been nearly impossible had it not been for those who took the time to care for me. Judy Divine e-mailed every few days with a few encouraging words or a scripture to hang on to when things were difficult. Those e-mails became a needed outlet for me to share day-to-day frustrations and doubts as well as victories. I did not realize then how important it was to have a place to vent; someone who would listen without criticizing or trying to give answers when there were none. Countless others wrote, called, and prayed faithfully for us. We are indebted to each.

Laughter became a vital part of our everyday life. I laughed when I would ordinarily have cried or become angry. I laughed even though I was so sick I wasn't sure I could make it through the day myself. I laughed while my heart ached over the Mom that was no longer there. And I learned first hand how to find the good in everything that happened.

If I stood Mother up to move her and she went to the bathroom all over the chair and floor, we laughed at the fact that we no longer had to worry about her bowels moving. "Can't complain, can we, Momma? This is what we wanted. Maybe not right here, not right now, but its okay isn't it?" We both would be giggling as I sat her down and began the task of cleaning her up. It would take some time to accomplish that task; often I would struggle to not throw up in the midst of it all. It was important that Mother not feel embarrassed or think she had done something wrong.

These accidents would sometimes happen when the kids or grandchildren were visiting. They would quietly excuse themselves while I restored order to the place and then they would return and continue the visit. I was always impressed by the kindness and understanding of others and pleased when they took time to hug Mom and reassure her of their love. Company other than family would generally go outside or to another room when I began to move her and then return when the coast was clear. I found most people to be sympathetic and loving in these circumstances and was surprised that I was not embarrassed.

Every morning before I got Mother out of bed I tried to get her laughing about something. "Morning, Sunshine! How is you today? Are you ready to cook my breakfast this morning?" "Russell is hungry and said you would come fix his breakfast for him. Is that okay?" "Let's go, girl! You is got work to do today!" "Morning, Sassafras! Is you a sassy woman today?" "Morning,

Sugar Lump! How is you this fine day?" I would poke her tummy, "You don't seem too sugary today, but you sure are a lumpy little gal!"

If silly chatter didn't get her to laughing, singing would. With long drawn out tones I would begin: "Good morning to you! Good morning to YOU! Good morning, dear Mommeee, good morning to-oo-oo you-uuu-uuu!" We would both giggle and then I would proceed to get her out of bed and onto the potty. There we would laugh and make plans for the day.

Mother had to take a fiber supplement twice a day. For awhile, the fiber crackers worked well; she could hold them herself and nibble on them while I took care of her. When she no longer would eat those crackers, I switched her to the liquid supplements. That was a challenge in itself. If she didn't get the stuff down right away, it would get so thick you could spoon it. The solution was for me to take some with her (not fun).

"Hey, Momma, here is our juice. Drink it right down for me." If she slowed down we would make a contest to see who could finish first. If it thickened before she got it all down, I had to add water. The fiber pills did not work at all so when she tired of the liquids we would go back to the crackers for awhile. She would never realize my constant struggle to know which way to give her the fiber supplement each day. She did know that we would always celebrate and rejoice over an empty glass or finished cracker.

Every day brought new challenges. We accepted the changes as *blessings to be unwrapped*. I celebrated everything with her. I took pictures of her constantly; many of which will mean absolutely nothing to anyone else and even may seem unnecessary. I am thankful I have those pictures now to help me relive some of the most cherished times of my life.

When Mother ended up on the floor, I took pictures of her "slumber parties". When she broke out all over with a rash, I took a picture of her big smile in the middle of that bright red face. I have pictures of her asleep holding a half eaten sandwich to her mouth. One favorite photo is her holding a spoon of food in mid-air while dozing off. When she awoke, she just continued to eat as if nothing had interrupted her meal. (You *can* believe it. I have pictures!)

I have photos of Mother reading her books and looking through her many cards. I am the only one who can look at the photos and hear the sweet sound of her voice as she read them. I alone can see her face

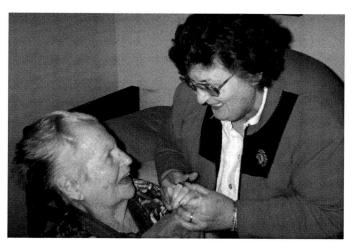

light up when we talked about the person who sent the card.

The month before Mother went to the hospital for the last time, Russell put a camera by his chair and snapped several pictures of Mother and me together. These are priceless to me. A particular favorite is her laughing as I trimmed her nails. We were absolutely silly; it helped keep things in perspective.

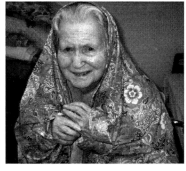

I have a great picture of one of the last times she dressed herself. I remember it well. I had gone into the closet to get her some shoes to match her dress. I had given her the dress to put on. "Momma, put your dress on while I get you some shoes to wear." When I returned, she had the dress on her head like a shawl and was holding it together under her chin.

"What are you doing, silly girl?" Mother gazed up at me with such an impish grin. She was enjoying her new venture.

"You little urchin! You are supposed to put that on your body, not your head!" It was clear to see that dressing herself was becoming a thing of the past. I soon began having her help me choose which outfit she wanted to wear. Then I dressed her and combed her hair.

"Ain't I pretty?" she would say as she patted her chest and held her little chin high in the air.

"Oh, Momma, you is beautiful today!"

Bedtime was always an event in our home. Usually Russell would be in his chair with his bare feet on the footrest. I would stand Mother up against her walker and we began our nightly journey. "Momma, go get those toes." Russell would wiggle his toes and she would take one step toward him. She would look at him and back at me.

She usually had to be coaxed each step of the way. Sometimes I would put an arm under hers and sing my version of the Rawhide theme song; "Movin,' movin' movin'! Get them feetsies movin'!" A few giggles and off we'd go; maybe two or three steps at a time. When we reached Russell's feet, I would try to get Momma to pull his toes. He would wiggle them and she would giggle and look at me as if to say "I don't think I should do that."

One evening, Mother and I were making the long trek to her bedroom when she suddenly pushed the walker away from her. Before I could stop her, she bent at the waist and had her hands on the floor in front of her. I gulped thinking she was falling only to relax when she raised back up with a piece of paper in her hand.

"Thank you, Tidy Muffin, for helping me keep the floor clean." And, thank God that she didn't turn over!

Those treasured moments of fun that we used

to make the long, slow trip to bed each night more bearable now serve as a comfort to me. Again, Russell captured some of it on film for us to share in years to come. Taking time with someone pays great dividends. We could never have shared these fun times in a care facility. We both sacrificed at times to make even a simple trip through the house special. It was important to both of us that Mother be able to go to bed knowing she was loved and cared for unconditionally.

Drawing her attention toward simple daily activities presented another challenge. I found the newspaper helpful in this area. Spreading the newspaper out on her lap, I would discuss the people in the pictures. No, I didn't know them any more than she did, but I could sure tell some great stories about them!

"Look, Momma, at that cute baby on the blanket! Let's *buy* one of those!" The ad, in beautiful color, displayed baby furniture and toys.

She took the paper, completely captivated by the little baby's picture.

"Tell Russell to go buy us a baby. We need one around here, don't we?" She looked at him, then at the picture. She loved babies; that was probably a happy thought for her.

Several times I let her help me with the grocery list. She looked at the pictures and would sometimes point to something, though that was a rare occurrence indeed.

It takes a lot of time and resolve to pull a loved one back into your world. It is definitely worth it. Quality of life is not so much a measure of what a person can or cannot do, as it is how that person is made to feel in their circumstances. There are many people up and about who are not made to feel loved and accepted by those around them.

Some of our best moments came unannounced as Mother was encouraged by someone to talk or to do some activity. An occupational therapist, Ginger Wimberly, and a speech therapist named Melissa were determined to get Mother talking at least enough to communicate with us. On one visit, they insisted I sit at the table to view their progress. I listened as one of them softly sang "*Mary had a Little Lamb*" to Mother as her eyes danced with glee. "This time, Geneva, you have to sing the words with us. On the count of three we will all begin. One, two, three," Melissa commanded and then began to sing. I heard my Mother singing softly with them. How long it had been since I heard her sing; how sweet the sound of her voice. I quickly scooted to the kitchen as the tears ran down my face.

Would she remember this experience tomorrow? Probably not, but who knows what had been stirred up deep inside her soul. The Bible teaches us that laughter and good thoughts are as good medicine to the soul. Perhaps this special time had healed yet another hurt of the past and prepared her more fully for that time when she could sing with the angels in the very presence of Jesus. And I had gained another precious memory to bank for later.

The occupational therapists would encourage

her to use her arms and hands in everyday tasks. Finding something for her to do became a game. While doing laundry I would fold clothes in her room so she could "help" me. It became Mother's job to fold wash cloths. It was a rare event to have even three or four of them folded properly, or folded in the same way. She would carefully fold one cloth corner to corner and then the next one would be folded up into a tiny square. Some were hardly touched at all and it became quite a messy stack when she was finished. It didn't matter at all; she always got a hug and a "thank you" from a daughter who was just glad to have her company.

She must have gotten tired and frustrated at her loss of mobility and motor skills, yet I was constantly amazed at her sweet, sweet disposition. I never grew weary watching her eat or rest or watch TV. She went to sleep often while eating, and I enjoyed watching the process. She had the softest, wrinkle free skin, and her eyes and lips seemed to smile even in sleep. It's a picture of contentment you cannot capture on film.

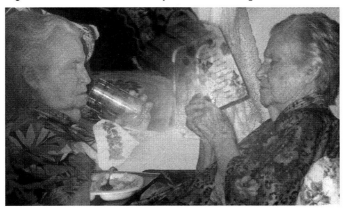

More than once she stopped at the day bed or piano to straighten something on her way to bed. She always paused at the mirror to gaze at the old woman there. That was my cue to coax a smile for her to see as she looked herself over. We all look better when we smile!

ENTHUSIASTIC ENCOURAGERS

*ow many bottles of perfume or hand lotion can an eighty year old woman use? Would she really want another pair of fluffy house slippers or a frilly gown to put into a drawer? Why keep sending cards when she probably doesn't even look at them? Besides what do you say week after week after week to someone who doesn't leave the house? Flowers too soon fade away and a plant would be one more thing for the caregiver to tend. How do you visit with someone who doesn't talk to you, someone you hardly know yourself? Do you just smile and nod as you pass by? Short-term illness is one thing but what do you do year-after-year to encourage someone?

In the years of caring for Mother I experienced the kindnesses and compassions of others in creative ways I had never anticipated. Mother took pleasure in each bottle of perfume or lotion or pair of slippers that was given to her. We appreciated those who cared enough to give. I always marveled at the many creative gifts she received such as an angel nightlight, figurine, tiny waterfall ceramic or a colorful notebook and pen.

During Mother's last four years with us, Russell's responsibilities as a director of missions included overseeing fourteen churches and being available to help their pastors when needed. As with all our ministries, he and I worked together as much as possible. Our home served as the associational office and I helped with the secretarial duties. This meant we had people from a number of our churches picking up projects or using the copier throughout the week. We encouraged them to come on in even when we were not home.

We strongly suggested that anyone stopping by, visit with Mother first and let her know who they were and what they were going to do. Many times we heard glowing reports of her reaction to their visits; sometimes she even gave a word or two in response, and always had a smile for anyone who spoke to her. Someone admonished us once to never say she didn't talk because "your mother speaks volumes with her eyes and beautiful smile."

And she truly did! When someone would pause to talk with her, her eyes began to dance. Her face would clearly tell the story; you knew you were doing a good thing. Sometimes behind the sunshine and bubbles was a momma that was being a little imp. She truly was a treasure!

Mother was always delighted when Helen and

Donna came to care for her or to visit. Helen Wall lived nearby and brought such joy when she arrived.

"Hi, Momma! How are you doing today? Are they being good to you?" She insisted her name and phone number be posted on Mom's bathroom mirror. Knowing Helen was available when needed made it much easier for us to leave Mother in the care of strangers. She proved she really was willing to come anytime when she got out of bed one night to come help us. Russell and I were having difficulty managing Mother in her weakened condition, and needed Helen's help to get her into bed safely.

When Donna Petersen came to help, she would first head straight to Mother's chair and wrap her arms around her. "Hi, Susie's Momma! You love me more than her, don't you?" Those two would snuggle and giggle awhile before we could visit. She wrote this thoughtful poem as a gift to us after watching Mother and I together.

My Caregiver

She wakes me every morning,
On her face a great big smile.
She asks me how I am today,
As she gets me started on my way.
Her touch is light,
Her voice is tender,
Her heart is full of love.
Her eyes are bright,
Her smile is sweet,

As she gets me on my feet.
Everyday, it's the same routine,
But she never complains, even tho' I do.
She does for me the things I use to do for her.
Don't know what I'd do without her,
She means so much to me.
I hope she knows how much I love her,
Since I can't tell her anymore.
She is my life, my care giver,
She is my daughter.

Often Russell scheduled committee meetings in our home so we wouldn't have to be gone late at night. People came in the front door, past Mom's chair and into the dining room to meet. We always made sure to introduce new people to her as they came in. Often Pastor Roger Easter and others would leave the table in the middle of the meeting to go visit her a few minutes. "Are you okay in here?" "Can you hear your television?" "Do you need more water?" How important and valued this must have made Mother feel.

One day I saw Gary and Cheri Klapp get out of their van with a huge picnic basket and a song book and I knew we were in for something special. Dressed for the occasion, Gary had on overalls and a plaid shirt and Cheri wore a print dress with a white eyelet collar.

"Hello, Geneva," Gary said. "Are you ready to go on a picnic?" Cheri spread a red checkered table cloth on Mother's tray as Gary unloaded the basket.

"Do you like fried chicken, Geneva?" quizzed

Cheri. It was a feast of chicken, mashed potatoes and all the trimmings (with leftovers for later). As we ate, they stood nearby and sang some country songs and old gospel hymns. It refreshed me just to watch Mother have so much fun. They could not know how much she enjoyed picnics, fried chicken, and good music. Their surprise visit was a home run for sure! Through pictures, we would relive that special occasion many times. Those church friends had decided I had missed too many of the fun events at church and Mother needed to be able to enjoy some of them as well. Instead of merely bringing us a plate of food, they brought us our own private picnic. What a treat!

I've come home to find dishes washed, Momma with a snack, or flowers on her table. One day I came home to find Thelbert Gott sitting in the chair next to Mom and both of them had their eyes peeled on the birdfeeders outside the front window. "Momma and I have been visiting about the birds," he said. Mother's eyes danced with excitement as Thelbert elaborated on the colorful goldfinch and cardinals they had seen. My mother, like her mother, loved the attention of the guys and she relished the visit of this new friend from one of our churches.

Being in the ministry, we were blessed to have music evangelists and preachers in our home from time to time. Mother clapped to the music when quadriplegic YoYo Collins filled the house with old familiar southern gospel tunes. When the Price Twins, Mark and Mead, brought their violins, they had Mother's full attention. Fair Play's youth group sang for her and practically hugged her to pieces. I marveled at the sweetness of each of these young people as she soaked it all in.

Native American Evangelist, C.W. Springwater, brought his entire family over just to sing a Navajo hymn for her, and I realized again that each of these folk were using all their time and talents for the Lord, and blessing us in the process. It reminded me that God is the One we serve as we care for others in whatever way He leads. "And whatsoever ye do in word or deed, do all in the name of the Lord Jesus, giving thanks to God and the Father by him" (Colossians 3:17 KJV).

> [1]*"Amazing Grace, How sweet the sound, that saved a wretch like me. I once was lost, but now am found, was blind but now I see."*

Texas musician Sam Craig sang the verse softly, with such feeling. Momma's beautiful eyes were glued to his smiling face as he continued. She absolutely beamed, and I knew that, in her heart at least, she was clapping and raising her hands in praise to her Lord.

> *"When we've been there 10,000 years, bright shining as the sun . . ."*

Now Sam was lifting his voice as though he was singing to the multitudes in a large crusade. A tear drifted down Momma's happy face. She knew he was singing about her eternal home.

What a blessed moment we were privileged to share. When I think of the many, many beautiful

Christian people growing sad and grouchy as they age, I begin to wonder. Are their souls merely starving for some word from Jesus? Perhaps after hearing Bible preaching and gospel singing all their lives, they now find themselves in a foreign realm with someone else making choices for them, often lacking the spiritual nourishment they need. We somehow must take care of the hungry souls of the elderly as well as their bodies. "God, help us care for them as You would!"

Another blessing for Mother was the many cards and letters she received. My brother's wife, Linda, could turn a small piece of card stock into a work of art by just adding a few stickers or pasting on some picture she cut from a magazine. A bit of her grandchild's art work or a photo of some beautiful flower gave us much to enjoy. She faithfully sent cards every week even as she faced terminal cancer herself. And, as for what to write week after week, Linda had the answer. She knew that news of Richard's latest fishing trip or a report on how many bags of leaves he gathered in a week would seem unexciting to some but not to his mother. She once wrote an entire card about watching a butterfly on a flower. As I re-read those cards to Mother, I could sense her being right there in the midst of the activity. I really think these cards did much to keep Mother connected with her past and with the world outside. In retrospect, the opportunity to create these cards was probably a great help to Linda in her last year.

Hearing from old friends stirred our hearts and reminded Mother of days gone by. Gary Crawford was such a friend. One of Richard's best buddies through all twelve years of school at Goodman, he practically lived at our house growing up. His letter to Mother on her 85th birthday has much to say about the value of friends and family.

> *Geneva,*
>
> *I'm so thankful for folks like you and your family. No telling where I would be without people like you, Frank, Richard, and Sue. Thanks for being there. A person can live a lifetime without realizing the influence they have had on others. I will always remember how faithful you were to provide for your family and the strays and for caring enough that we lived the right way. Most of all I'm very pleased to read of your Christianity and work in the Church. God Bless.*
>
> *Have a Happy Birthday.*
>
> *With Love,*
>
> *Gary L. Crawford, A Stray*

Mother's childhood and young adult years as well as her early married life had been very difficult. Even with prodding she would tell us very little about those periods except for a few years in her twenties. During that time, she was governess for the Oven family in Enid, Oklahoma. She told of how she loved and cared for those children and how their mother was more like a sister to her than an employer. Trips with the family took her to places she had only dreamed about. She would sit tall as she spoke and I could envision her as the prim and proper red-haired servant girl with all the social graces required for the task.

I had dreamed of locating the family for her one day. Miraculously, my brother, Richard's work transferred him to Enid. While there, his wife, Linda, located the Oven family home. She also found Mary, who had been the family cook when Mother was working for the Ovens. Linda helped an elderly Mary make an audio tape for Mom. She also got permission to photograph the outside of the house and the grounds that had been such a special part of Mom's young life. Watching Linda and Mother go through the little album filled with photos and seeing Mom relive precious times was a dream come true. That album would stay on Mother's table for many years for her to enjoy. I would often find her asleep with it in her hand. God had richly blessed all of us with more than I dared to ask. And there was more to come.

Linda had found the address of Joan, one of the Oven children. After writing to her, asking if she remembered her former governess, we awaited a reply. Mother was on the edge of her chair as she read the letter from her dear "Joanie". Just listen to the extra treasure Joan included with the letter:

Dear Susie and Geneva,

Of course I remember "Nursie"!

The enclosed copy is part of a composition I wrote for English class in 1949.

It's as if I had written it yesterday. . . . much love to you all,

Joan (Oven) Bent

The composition talked of the Oven home:

One thing which remains so vividly in my mind is the big, brown bed where our beloved red-haired nurse, Geneva ("Nursie" to me) slept. Geneva shared the room with Mary, the cook (that was in the pre-war days, when nurses and cooks were plentiful). Mother decided it would be a better arrangement if Geneva would sleep in the nursery and could be nearer us. Well, to get back to the bed, its slats had a terrible habit of falling when an over-abundance of pressure was placed on it, and you can imagine how our shrieks of childish glee would fill the room when poor, tired Geneva, who was, shall we say, pleasingly plump, would wearily sink to the bed and . . . crash! There she would be, sprawled on the mattress, one side of which would have fallen on the floor and the other side still on the bed, and her feet hanging over the side board, her face half filled with disgust and half with surprise.

At the time we got the letter, Mother was able to read it herself, and to answer it. She repeated several paragraphs and rambled a lot as she would write a spell, then doze, then write some more. I sent the letter, just as she had written it to Joan. Mother was so pleased to write her. I did not think it had to be perfectly written; it clearly was from her heart to a little girl she had loved and cared for. It was to be the last letter she was able to write.

We laughed and laughed at the story of the slats falling as we recalled incidents in our own home of that very thing. I reminded Mother how much Joan must have loved her to include her in that beautiful story she had written so many years ago.

I saw a tear as she replied, "I loved those children so much."

That simple little letter gave us countless moments of sharing through the years that were to follow; just one good memory of her past that we could now enjoy afresh.

Going the extra mile like these folk and many others did meant putting others' needs ahead of their own. It meant risking embarrassment in order to help someone else feel loved and wanted. I do realize it is hard to talk with someone when they can't return the conversation. We often don't know what to say. Sometimes we are simply unsure of what their response, if any, will be. For me it is worth the chance just to bring a smile to a lonely face.

Many times I have visited homes where an elderly person would be in the room and I really did not pay attention to them. If the hostess did not introduce us, I found it easy to walk past them without lingering. That was before we had Momma. How sorry I am for ever ignoring anyone, especially a homebound older person. Watching Mother react when someone paid attention to her has made me realize how important it is to treat them like the person they are with all the honor and respect they are due. A simple smile or pat on the hand does wonders for a lonely soul. Now, whether introduced or not, I go to that person first and let them know that they still have value and that I am glad to see them.

I saw a lady walk right past her friends in town because one of the friends had some form of memory loss. Not knowing what to say or how to communicate, the woman simply chose to walk by quickly with a simple nod. Sometimes in these situations, the "normal" person might get warm hugs and conversation while their mate, whose mind isn't as sharp as it used to be, is completely ignored and left standing alone. This is hard on everyone. How sad.

People walk in and out of our lives and each leaves a mark. How great it is to be able to share with others how they've touched our lives in some way. No good memory is too small to share with a lonely person. No card is too plain if it's filled with personal accounts of love and caring. No smile, pat on the hand or spoken word is ever wasted on a man, woman or child in need of encouragement. How easy it is to change a life; how little time it really takes to be a friend to someone.

REMARKABLE RELATIONSHIPS

⌒

One of my greatest encouragers while I cared for my mother was my dear husband, Russell. He was there each and every time I needed him. He was always ready to help physically, emotionally, spiritually. He carefully guided me through each decision, but always let me make the final call. He is a good husband and friend to me and was a great son-in-law to my mother. His attitude toward her was always one of respect and honor; he had a tenderness and understanding that I did not always have.

After our children had grown and left the house, Russell and I had enjoyed many years with just the two of us. My mother had taught me, "Take good care of your husband, and he will take good care of you." Well, I spoiled him rotten and he returned the favor! We were a team. We enjoyed doing things for one another, holding hands, and simply being together.

When he came home from town, it was my practice to stop whatever I was doing, give him a hug, and spend time sharing even the most routine details of my day. We planned long trips to visit family and friends. With Russell being a pastor, we went to every convention, retreat, or learning event connected with our church and denomination that we could. Many of these trips meant being out of town three or four days at a time. Last minute get-togethers with friends were no problem for us. Our office was in our home so we had the freedom to change our schedules and be gone almost any day we chose.

For the first few years with Mother, not much of that changed. She was able to take care of many of her own needs and did not need the constant care she would later require. Russell had a busy schedule as pastor of the church in Fair Play during that time. His full work week made the transition to living with Mother easier for both of us. Then ever so gradually, Mother became my main focus; her needs were immediate regardless of any other. I could no longer just stop when he came home and give attention to his needs. The couch in the living room would often become my bed as I sensed the need to get up frequently to check on her. Did I hear her coughing? Was she sleeping okay? Was she cool enough? Did she need more covers?

There were times when I had to work hard to not allow resentment to build. After all those years of doing everything together, I did not like sending him off to a meeting by himself. There were times when he would choose to sit with Mother so that I could get away for a few hours. It soon became necessary to be more selective with our schedules and focus on Mother and her needs. We knew we would not always have her with us. Open and honest communication served as our best resource.

Our happy-go-lucky lifestyle soon became much more confined and structured. This was very difficult for me. My stubborn will got in the way. Deep down I wanted things as they were without all these interruptions in our comfortable schedule. I wanted Mom to be here for sure, but I wanted the rest of our lives to stay the same. Life does not stay the same. There are always changes when we have parents, kids, grandkids, and other family move in and out of our lives seeking love and nurturing.

It had always been our habit to go to bed at the same time. Russell and I would hold hands and have prayer together, then reflect on the day's activities. There was nothing the world hurled our way that could penetrate the peace I felt as I went to sleep in my husband's arms after reviewing the goodness of God in our daily lives.

In the early days of caring for Mother, Russell patiently waited each night for me to get Mother to bed before he headed for our bedroom. When she was maneuvering on her own, it didn't take long for her to be tucked in for the night. Then, as she began to need more help, he would go to bed alone.

The last few years, putting Mother to bed took

about an hour. It was a long, slow trip from her chair to the bedroom. It took time for her to use the commode, and to get her cleaned up and dressed for bed. Sometimes I would be so tired and sleepy, that I would grow impatient coaxing her to take her meds and finish her drink. Many times I would have her all tucked in and be heading for my bed when familiar sounds would tell me that I had a Momma to clean up again, and a bed to change before I could retire.

I would chatter with her as I got her clean and comfy once more. "Whatcha doin,' Girl? Think I needed something to do? Too early for bed, eh?" These were the times I knew for certain that people were praying for us.

I was always amazed at Russell's patience. There were nights when I know he was ready for bed long before we were, but he would stay in his chair, wiggling his toes to encourage Mother to walk another step. I wondered if he ever wanted to say, "Just put your mother in that wheel chair and get her to bed." I probably would have more than once; he never did. I would use the wheelchair when it was necessary, and let Russell go on to bed, while I cared for her. I often had to awaken him to come help me, especially if I could not get her to turn around and sit on the bed.

At first this was difficult for me. I am, like my mother, a self-sufficient doer. I didn't think I needed any help. I did not want to put anyone else out, especially Russell. It was, after all, *my* mother and therefore, *my* responsibility. Time took its toll on that theory as did my outspoken husband. In kind, gentle ways he helped me see that as we became one, she became *our* mother and *our* responsibility together. I learned to ask for help even when I felt sure I could handle things on my own.

At the last, we went through a long period of time when it took both of us to put her to bed. She could not seem to figure out how to turn around to the bed and sit on it. We talked with the healthcare workers, especially the physical therapists. While they offered several ideas for equipment that might be helpful, we found none that really suited our needs.

Finally, we came up with a workable solution that would be easy for us and safe for her. Russell pushed her into the bedroom in her wheelchair, and I put her walker in front of her. I helped her stand up to the walker while he quickly moved the wheelchair and put her commode in its place. With everything in place, I could usually get her diaper down and set her on the commode by myself.

When she was through with the bathroom, and I had her dressed for bed, I called him back. Again we stood her up against the walker while he moved the commode. Since she would not, or could not turn around to the bed, Russell moved a small, swivel desk chair under her. We swiveled her around to where her back was to the bed. Putting the walker in front of her, we stood her up yet again and Russell moved the swivel chair out of the way. She was now standing, facing away from the bed and about a foot from it. With one of us on either side of her, we each kept one hand on her back while we used the free hand to pull the hospital bed up to her bottom. She could then sit down on the edge of the bed, and I could finish from there.

There were times when I longed to just go sit on the deck with Russell and visit about the day's events. I missed the free time to just hang out together awhile, or have a spur-of-the-moment picnic or some such. He never complained, but I am sure he missed our privacy and having his meals on time. He worried about my needs as well.

An occasional nap was usually out of the question. It seemed there was a constant flow of activity on just the day we yearned to slip away and rest. If it wasn't a healthcare worker coming in or leaving, it was the telephone, or time to do something for Mother. We were blessed with flexible work schedules. Often late into the night he would study and I would catch up on office work.

It eventually became apparent that we simply must plan one day a week for the two of us to get away. We worked hard to schedule help on Thursday of each week and made plans to go somewhere together. For me, these were "dates" with my favorite guy, and I looked forward to them as much as I did when we were courting. Most often our trips were simply to a nearby town for a meal and a walk through the mall or downtown square. We enjoyed going for a leisurely drive, stopping along the way as some store or garage sale caught our eye. Knowing we had this day to plan on, we could schedule outings with friends as well.

If the weather was bad or we just didn't want to go somewhere, we planned activities for the two of us at home. We needed to again schedule regular time away each week because we otherwise did not take time to refresh and to simply enjoy one another's company as we should.

Only in looking back, do I realize what a toll caring for Mother took on our relationship. I can say with complete confidence that neither Russell nor I would have done anything differently. We feel it was not only our responsibility to care for her but also our honor and our privilege. While we did make some sacrifices, we were indeed blessed as a result of those years with her.

For those who are reading this book, have you considered what others are going through as they care for a loved one? Is there some way you might lift their load? If you cannot help in the actual caring for someone, get creative and find something you *can* do. Do you need to help support financially? Maybe you could hire someone to sit with the loved one so the caregivers could take a day away. Consider having a pizza or meal delivered to the home; what a welcome surprise that would be. Could you go visit, or send flowers *to the caregiver?* For us, it was amazing what a simple phone call from one of our children would do to lift our spirits on a tiring day.

With Mother living with us, family often gathered in our home for the holidays. It was a challenge to get Mother up to the dining table so she could eat with us. Her wheelchair was big and bulky, and we could not get it close enough to the table for her to eat comfortably. Mother was too cautious to ever turn loose of her walker long enough for me to move it out of the way so she could turn around. When it was obvious that Mother could no longer come to the dining table, I would give her lunch in her recliner in the living room. This meant I had my meal there, too, so she would not be alone.

One Thanksgiving I decided we should all have a meal at the table together, and I was determined to make it happen. My brother Richard, and his wife Linda, were home for the holidays and my cousin Penny and her husband Bud, had joined us for the feast.

Instead of having Mother walk into the living room as usual, I turned her, walker and all, toward the dining room. A surprised family looked on as I had her walk forward until the walker was hitting the table. When she was as close as possible, I pushed a dining chair under her bottom and guided her to sit down. Now, I could fold the walker up and move it out of her way.

"Grab that table," I instructed my onlookers. "Move it right up to her so she can enjoy the meal with us." What a meal indeed! Our table was practically in the living room, but no one cared. As Mother listened to the tales, I wondered if she recalled family gatherings of the past. I knew for sure this would not be the last time she could sit at our table. I would be more careful to find ways to move things so she could be part of the activity and not be left in another room by herself.

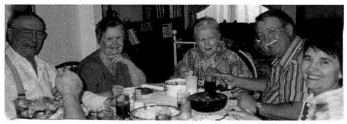

Bud   Penny   Mother   Richard   Linda

It wasn't possible for us to spend as much time with our children as we wanted. Caring for Mother took time and was the priority, especially in her last years. The children were loving and respectful to her and to us; always ready to rearrange their schedules when possible to accommodate our needs. We did miss the freedom to go to their homes to visit as much as we wanted.

Our five grandchildren were each one a very special delight to their great-grandmother. Her smile would broaden as the two older boys, Jeremy and Allen, would enter the room. They will never know how much their hugs and chatter would mean to a feeble old woman. I'm sure that I am not partial when I say they are both handsome young men. She would have agreed with me if she could speak; I am sure that sparkle in her eye and broad smile let them know they were precious to her.

Melanie loved to massage "Gram's" fingers. She would stand by her chair as long as Mother would hold on, all the while telling her she was so sweet and how much she loved her.

Younger Melissa stayed in our home during Vacation Bible School each summer so she and Mother had a real bond. From the very beginning, Melissa would find her place nearest Grandma's chair. "Grandma Geneva, I'll get you a blanket for your feet," she would say as she set out to make her great-grandmother comfortable. The two of them spent many hours reading their books while grinning and winking at each other.

Rusty was the youngest (and, of course, also a handsome young man). He hardly knew Grandma when she wasn't feeble. It became his self-appointed mission to see to her every need, especially food and drink. He insisted on taking her meals to her and cleared her dishes away when she was finished. Grandma really looked forward to all the special attention that she knew she would get when Rusty came to spend a week each summer.

Each great-grandchild was careful to greet her upon arriving and hug and kiss her before leaving. Their presence and attention filled her mind with happy thoughts to give purpose and meaning to another day. When I look back on the pictures of our family and notice how often a child is snuggled next to their grandparent, I get a new understanding of how precious little children were to Jesus. Oh, to have a pure heart like these little ones.

Their parents, our four children, also gave of themselves each time they visited. Debbie worked in the healthcare field, and was quick to let me know of any concerns she may have had about her grandmother's health and well being. It was helpful for me to have her to rely on when I had a medical question. Our younger daughter, Laura, played the piano for Mother and talked with her about everything. Her experiences working with young children were quite helpful. She suggested great ideas to keep Mother occupied. She also bought us a cell phone so we could get out of the house for a few hours and have peace knowing caregivers could reach us if need be. Our sons, Michael and Ricky, enjoyed doting on Grandmother. They brought her candy and gifts and talked of old times with her. We relied heavily on our boys when we needed something moved or repaired. They also surprised us one Christmas with satellite TV and a DVD player the next year so we could have wholesome programs and movies to watch.

Younger people have so much to give to older ones. A little time and a smile can do much to ease life for a shut-in, and give the caregiver a little break in the everyday routine. How thankful I am for our family and their care for one another. Our family is somewhat unique. Russell and his first wife had fostered Debbie from the age of ten and had adopted Michael at age four and Laura at birth. My first husband and I had taken in Ricky and raised him as our son from the age of nine. When our respective mates died and Russell and I met, Ricky and Debbie were grown but Michael and Laura were only eleven and ten. It could only have been God who blended this family of ragamuffins together so beautifully. Their visits were a constant reminder of the importance and the strength of family.

The lives of our younger generation are enriched by spending time with older people. What a shame that we often get so busy filling our lives with activities that we neglect building healthy relationships. Granddaughter Melissa was in her early teens when she wrote this letter to Mother.

> *Dear Grandma,*
>
> *I love you a lot and I always will! You are the best and you are very funny. You always make me laugh and giggle! You are very nice to me and thank you for saying good things about me. I really love you very much.*

Who knows how much Mother's positive, loving compliments helped a young teen girl feel good about herself. Mother living in our home just naturally brought us all together more often than if she hadn't lived with us. Having Mother with us was a good thing for our entire family.

Michael came to see Grandma several times in the hospital. He was eleven when I married his dad and I often said he was happier to get "a real live Grandma" than anything else. On his last visit with her, Mother really looked him over as he came in; there was a faint smile on her face. Then, as she dozed off, he just rubbed her shoulders for the longest time, gently kissed her forehead, and left the room. We sat in the outer room and cried together realizing how great our loss would be.

I don't think he could realize how short her time was until he saw her in that hospital bed. It is so important that the truth of a family member's condition be told to all the family. They need the opportunity, when possible, to visit with their loved ones. Our children knew Grandma was going to heaven and that she was ready for the journey. They were assured that we had done all we could do here. It was simply time for her to go.

It is my sincere belief that our children and grandchildren knew as we did that caring for Mother was God's gift to our family. He had entrusted us with His child to love and care for in her time of need. I'm proud of each of them and pray for them and their families that God will provide in their times of need. They have truly done as the Scripture says, "Honor your father and mother, that you may have a long, good life . . ." (Exodus 20:12a TLB).

In a very real sense, the relationships in a caregiver's life are strained daily. Interactions among family members are not the same as they were; lack of time, energy, and availability take their toll on even the strongest of ties. This, for some, is the only view they can see.

Personally, I choose the other side of the coin. Yes, it was hard. Yes, we made sacrifices. Yes, the old familiar gave way to the new and strange. But each of our lives was enriched as we gave of ourselves. We were touched by God's grace in a way we never could have known otherwise. The bond between us and those who stood with us is stronger than ever. We all have a renewed compassion for others and a fresh sense of well being within ourselves. To God be the glory, great things He has done!

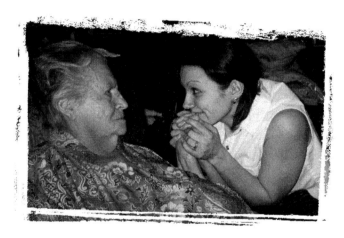

Mom-to-be Melanie massaging Gram's fingers

Richard's son Andy getting Lamp
Grandma made him

Grandma enjoying Laura and a
sleeping Rusty

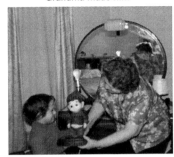

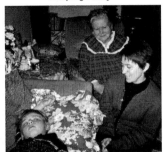

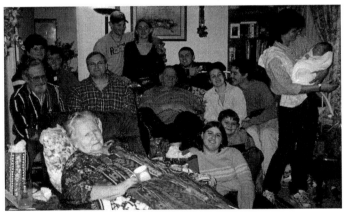

Proud Matriarch with grandchildren, great-grandchildren
and first great-great-grandchild

HEALTHCARE HEARTACHES

⌒

*T*he hospital and health care facilities generally proved to be a safe haven for Mother, a place for her to get good care, as well as a place for me to get a much-needed rest from the daily responsibilities of decision making. There were professionals there who knew how to care for Mother; they would understand better than I, what was happening with her waning health.

I am thankful for such institutions. I cannot count the times that we were in and out of the emergency room, hospital, and nursing homes with Mother during her eight years with us. After a few good months, or even a year, some illness would flare up that required more care than I could give at home.

I had a lot of confidence in Mother's primary care physician; he is one reason we chose to stay in the area when we searched for a home. When she came to

live with us, Mother had many physical needs, some
not so obvious. Her little ankles were swollen tight;
her digestive system was out of sync; her mobility was
impaired; her medications needed changing. From
the very first, Dr. Ronald Evans was dealing with an
older lady who could not communicate too well, and a
daughter who was unfamiliar with her mother's health
history.

Dr. Evans had a remarkable sensitivity to
Mother's needs. He was always patient with my endless
(too often repeated) questions, whether on the phone
or in the office. I appreciated the fact that he generally addressed his conversation to her, as his patient.
I do believe he recognized long before I did that her
answers and comments were not always reliable. How
very complicated it must be to care for someone under
those circumstances.

Over a period of eight years, Mother had many
other good medical doctors and surgeons caring for
her as well as some great nurses and aides. Many would
look her up just to enjoy her pretty smile. She delighted
in the special attention. Some would check often to see
if her legs were elevated properly, if she was covered up,
whether she needed some fresh water, a bag emptied,
or some other task done. They took the time to see that
she really did eat all her food or drink her liquids. They
were kind and gentle and caring. They treated her as a
person of value.

Mother was an easy patient. On one occasion,
she literally comforted the doctor and nurse when a

procedure caused her pain. Later I came to realize she would also tell them she was okay or that she had gone to the bathroom or whatever she needed to say to please them. Observing these things made me realize how difficult it must be to care for older patients you do not personally know.

The first few years when Mother was communicating well were understandably a little easier for everyone. She could respond to questions, express her pain and her discomfort. But even then, I soon learned that I had to keep a watchful eye. Family and caregivers must remain involved with the patient's care even in the hospital or nursing home. Someone who knows about the patient and their particular needs will help the transition go smoother. A loved one will understandably never get the quality of personal care somewhere else as they will at home, but personal involvement can help the health care workers as well as the patient.

There are skilled health care men and women who have a tender heart for those in their care, while others obviously work merely for wages. I've watched aides cleaning dirty bodies and beds, and marveled at their care and compassion. One housekeeper said, "I look on my job as a ministry. Even cleaning the floors is a way for me to help someone else." Persons with this attitude always make everyone's life easier and more enjoyable regardless of surrounding conditions.

No matter how great a hospital or nursing home seems to be, we must remember that they are staffed with real people. Whether we like it or not, people will make mistakes. Because of the nature of their jobs, however, those employed in health care jobs must be held to higher standards. While Mother's overall care was good, I did have some experiences that were quite disturbing.

I took care to weigh the issues that weren't really worth worrying over and tried not to be overly protective. However, when I walked into Mother's room one day and found her uncovered and naked from waist down, I was more than a little upset. Another day when I saw her in the lunchroom, her wheelchair in a puddle of urine and her hands full of mashed potatoes and gravy, I was crushed. Stripped of all dignity, she looked so helpless. I saw an aide start to take her plate, still full of food that no one had helped her to eat; and my heart ached to bring her back home.

One night I had to force myself to go out the door. I was leaving Mother in the care of two unkempt, shabbily dressed men; one in particular seemed to have been dragged in right off the streets. Thoughts of those two caring for that sweet old lady in the middle of the night sent chills up my spine. Would they be good to her? Would she be frightened? Would she understand when those big men were in her room at night?

We are taught in the business world that first impressions do make a big difference. Like it or not, we assume well-groomed, neatly dressed individuals will provide the best service. I think the same should even be more apparent in the healthcare field. It seems that individuals who care about themselves and their appearance would more likely care about their patients' well being. The two scruffy looking men in Mother's room could have been very qualified, kind, gentle workers who were there because they really cared for people and loved their jobs. However, that was definitely not my first impression.

Knowing how busy and short-handed the healthcare facility seemed to be, I rarely phoned them. When I did, often the person on the other end was brief or even rude, and clearly made me feel like an intruder. During one phone call when a nurse abruptly told me, "I guess she is doing okay today," I attempted to ask him to be more specific. Without even listening to my question, he replied; "I'm sure everything is okay here, thanks for calling," and hung up the phone. I dropped into the chair beside me with my mouth open and my heart pounding. If you are reading this and thinking it can't happen to you, check again. This was not some second-rate facility around the corner. And if you are a health care worker, please treat everyone including those on the telephone with respect and courtesy regardless of how busy or preoccupied you happen to be at the moment.

Doctors and nurses would tell me to stay home and get some rest myself. They tried to encourage me by saying she was getting good care, and I needed a break myself. I knew Mother's physical needs for the most part would be met, but I was more concerned about her emotional well being. Her surroundings were not like home and often the activity around her could be confusing or frightening.

On one visit, for instance, the lady in the next bed was obviously dying. Her daughter and family were there, holding her hand and crying. It was like a scene from a movie with all the sadness and grief you could picture. And there, in the bed next to the dying woman, was my Mother clinging to her blankets; the curtain between their beds was wide open revealing all the action on the other half of the room. This should not be. Couldn't someone along the way have shown a little compassion and turned Mother to the window? At the very least they could have pulled the curtain and turned her television on a low volume to distract her thinking. One patient does not need to watch another die and be carried out the door.

Mother was moved seven times over a period of a few months from the emergency room to the hospital, to the care facility, back to the hospital, to ICU, etc. With each move came challenges to face and more decisions to make. Each move also meant more needles in her deteriorating veins and bruised arms. Hopes would rise as she improved only to plummet when another issue surfaced.

After one of her many transfers, I found Mother was now getting oxygen. The nurse said that she had probably been given oxygen while being sent over from the hospital, and it had been left on her. She looked so uncomfortable and was tugging at the hose on her nose and ears. With my eyes tightly closed, I tried to picture myself in that bed. I listened to the sound of the noisy machinery and thought about that hose in my nose, tight over my ears, and snug under my chin. Would that be comfortable? No. Would I be happy? No. If those were my primary goals for Mother, I had to find out if the oxygen was an absolute necessity for her physical health.

After the nurse confirmed that the doctor had not ordered the oxygen, I took the hose gently from her face and she smiled. "Mommy, is that better? Is it okay if we just keep it off awhile?" Big smile. The nurse assured me that she would put it back on Mother if her oxygen level got too low, but for now she would be okay without it. Maybe she can rest a little. Maybe she will be less nervous, less worried. Maybe she'll begin to feel normal and well. Maybe.

One of my main concerns with elderly in the hospitals and nursing homes is their bowel movements. Many of mother's generation are laxative dependent. Couple that with inactivity and change of diet and you have big problems. Often I would work for days to get Mother cleaned out after a hospital stay, particularly in the first few years. When she would strain with no re-sults I would grab the Fleet Enema and suppositories and pour down liquids and fiber supplements.

Because I was so aware of Mother's needs, I would often inquire at the hospital or care facility about her bowel movements, especially if she was go-ing to be there more than one or two days. Someone would check the chart.

"She had one today."

"How do you know?"

"It is noted on the chart that she said she went to the bathroom early."

"Mother can't get out of bed on her own. If an aide didn't take her, she didn't go."

There were times when someone would try to convince me of their concern that Mother would become laxative dependent. For as long as I can remember, she took a laxative every day and now we had added a fiber supplement. She *was* laxative dependent and it was a little late to try to change it. When told she didn't need a laxative today, I would have to go back and tell them she had to have her laxatives every single day. Finally the doctor prescribed them for her and that made it official. I still had to check quite often to make sure they followed his orders.

My heart goes out to good health care personnel who write orders only to have them ignored. When Mother was choking on liquids, the kitchen staff had printed instructions to follow. All liquids, including water, were to be thickened. All foods were to be pureed. They were to send no straws or forks and to put her pureed food and thickened liquids in cups with handles so she could feed herself safely. Did it happen? Quite often it did not. Glasses of tap water and thin juices were often sitting right next to the bottle of thickener on her table. Even with printed instructions in plain sight, I found her chewing on a fork, poking a straw up her nose, and strangling on liquids.

It is so important, if you have loved ones in any care facility, to make unannounced visits. I rarely came at the same time of day to visit Mother. It was the only way that I could see how she was really being cared for. I should have been able to walk into her room at any time and find her in good hands. That was not always the case and it hurt to know I could not do anything about it.

The smallest things can make such a difference to both the patient and the family and friends. We all seem to do better in cheerful surroundings, especially those who are ill and lonely. A drab gray wall with a picture of one big piece of fruit or a single bloom is not comforting at all. If I had to stare at the same wall day after day, I would want something to turn my thinking to more pleasant times. When there were pictures of children at play, animals, or beautiful scenery, Mother seemed much more at ease. Those rooms not only cheered her, but they gave me something to talk about with her; they spurred happy thoughts and healthier hearts.

Like many people, I used to judge those who stuck their folks in a nursing home. "How could they do that? Don't they care?" I often thought that was just an easy way out for them. Just put them away and forget them. It is a fact that too many people do that very thing. For many, though, it's a difficult choice that had to be made, due to the caregiver's own health, work or other considerations. Now I realize for the first time how very hard it is to walk away and leave a loved one's care in a stranger's hands. I know how a heart breaks each time they look at you with saddened eyes as you go out the door leaving them behind. I have a friend who has had both her mother and her mother-in-law in an Alzheimer's unit for years. I know many others who have parents or mates in extended care facilities. It hurts to watch those we love deteriorate and not to be able to help them. The hurt deepens each time you walk away helpless to change the situation.

Sometimes it hurts even more to stay at home. From my journal just a few weeks before Mother died:

> *I am making myself not go to the hospital this morning. There are things I absolutely must do here, family chores as well as business to take care of. No one else can do them for me, but I want to leave it all undone and go to the hospital and hold my mother's hand. Somehow, I must let her go. While in her bedroom, I close my eyes and smell her fragrance. My fingers run slowly across the back of her chair as if hoping to touch her; to be able to cradle her in my arms once more. She is not there. Tears flow freely as I seek God's peace and strength to carry on without her!*

I want to honor every child, parent, and spouse whose care is consistent and whose heartache, unbearable at times, is real. I want to remind you that God sees and God cares. Your loved one may not respond in a way you can understand, but I know from caring for Mother, they do know you are there. Every touch of your hand, gentle kiss, or smile lets them know they are very much loved and are not forgotten.

Many times I wanted to gather her up in my arms and take her home. This was too hard. Walking out each day just tore me up. I would always give her a big smile and hug her and say everything would be okay. "They'll make you well soon and you can come home. Would you like that?" Big smiles of approval followed. But I couldn't know she would be okay and I didn't know if she would ever come home again.

During one long stay, Mother had gone from the hospital to the extended care facility and back to the hospital when I noticed her body begin to swell, especially her arms. I was assured this was probably her IV leaking or the huge amount of antibiotics she was taking, and it would be checked. The problem persisted but no one seemed to have an answer or even to be overly concerned.

Soon Mother was moved to the care facility again. She kept swelling and now her entire body was filled with fluids. Her elbows would quiver like jello when touched; her ankles, legs and toes were once again swollen and reddened. At first, I had wrongly concluded that her body was just shutting down and we were losing her. I didn't really know what to expect when someone may be dying.

Finally, in desperation, I asked to see her medicine chart and learned that they had not been giving her furosemide (Lasix). She had been on 160mg a day when she was originally admitted to the hospital.

"Why isn't she getting her water pill? Didn't someone notice it was left off her chart?" Further investigation showed that it was not on the chart when they transferred her to the health care facility the first time. Apparently some medicines were omitted in the transfer, perhaps a second medicine sheet was overlooked or something. That meant that the last several moves were without proper medicine. It was the weekend, but they assured me that they would get it started promptly Monday morning. I kindly suggested they get it today, and informed them that I would stay right there until it was done.

It was a few days later when I asked to see Mother's chart again because something was still not right. Sure enough there was no potassium ordered. Until I had Mother to care for, my knowledge of the effects of certain medicines had been limited to aspirin and cough syrup. By this time, however, I knew that when water pills were being taken, potassium was a must. By now my calm nature was outraged and I was much too angry to have a reasonable conversation. I wrote the administrator. I yelled at the doctors and nurses. "Doesn't anyone around here have any common sense? Don't you think if somebody is filling with fluid you should check the patient's medicine list? Not just what was prescribed originally, but what they are actually being given right now? Shouldn't you automatically check the potassium, too? Didn't all those blood tests you drew from her tell you anything?"

Another challenging time was trying medicines for Mother's dementia. Some of the medicines seemed to make her nervous. I wondered if she was beginning to realize too much of what was happening to her mentally and physically, and was unhappy about her circumstances. I had no way of knowing for sure. Those medicines are so strong and hard to predict. At one point I entered the nursing home to find her body jerking, and Mother was reaching for the sky while mumbling and groaning. I asked the doctor to take her off the medicines. "Mother is 90 years old," I told him. "She will never be what she used to be and I know I will not have her here forever. I want her life to be comfortable and happy and right now she is neither."

The medicines for dementia and Alzheimer 's disease often can do so much to help someone maintain a more normal life. Many of them have varying side effects and our bodies take a long time to adjust to them. If I would have let them keep her on those medications for a longer period of time, or try a different medication, maybe Mother would have eventually settled down some and even been able to communicate. But, was it really worth it? Did she need the added trauma? Did we? Here again is one of those instances where you make the best choice you can, and live with it.

There surely was some way I could have been better informed of possible consequences when asked to make decisions for her. I often felt like a first grader trying to pass a high school exam. Both Mother's physician and mine were very good to help keep me informed of her changes. They took the time to answer my questions, but I really didn't even know what questions to ask. By the time I figured out what I needed to know, she would be moved again, or another doctor would be on call. Sometimes I searched desperately for a nurse or aide that was personally familiar with her condition.

Maybe we should have considered more carefully the whole picture before we put Mother through some of the things we did. So many decisions frequently needed to be made without delay. Hospital staff, while polite, often seemed too busy to really explain things so I could understand. Isn't it interesting how simple a solution seems to be when it doesn't involve you or your loved one personally? Looking back I realize we could have more fully considered her age, her overall health needs, some specific health issues, and what quality of life she would have after the procedure or a particular form of therapy. Would I have changed my thinking? I think perhaps.

I wonder how families manage when there is no one to help them. What about the elderly couples with no children nearby, or the many folks who cannot read or comprehend what they are reading? How terribly confusing this must be for them, and how difficult for the hospital staff when so much is unknown about the patient.

I recall the first time I reckoned with the

thoughts of what was on the health care directive we had completed during Mother's first hospital visit. I was weary then and not ready to think of her life ending anytime soon even though I knew it was to be expected. Mother did not want any machines at all hooked up to keep her alive. But my heart raced as I wondered if the Do-Not-Resuscitate order on her bed applied if she choked on some food. Would they help her or just let her choke? The doctor was very patient with me and assured me that they would not just stand by and let her choke on her food. His assurance made me comfortable with the instructions she had left, but I'll not soon forget the initial panic I felt.

Looking back I realize many uninformed decisions can be made when filling out those directives. I've been quick to say "no machines hooked to me." I still feel that way and am comfortable with the decisions we made with Mother. I do wish I had taken time to become more familiar with the options available. It is not always simple to know where to draw the line; it's not always cut and dried. You need to consider what kind of resuscitation the patient wants, if any. Is the procedure to be used to prolong life or used only when needed to make the patient more comfortable and breathe easier while nature takes its course? And who is to make those decisions? A doctor? A trusted individual? All these things need to be specified in a health care directive.

It is so easy to take things for granted. After giving a copy of the Durable Power of Attorney and

Health Care Directive to the hospital and to the health care facility, I was assured there was no further need of concern on my part. This information would now become a permanent part of her records and readily available when needed. I was later surprised when a surgeon told me to verify that it was on record before her surgery. He said, "You must always ask to see the directive each time she is admitted so you can know for sure they do have it." Following his advice, I did check and it was nowhere to be found in her records. We immediately made duplicate copies for both vehicles and my purse and, from that time on, gave a copy to the attendant every time she was admitted or re-admitted to a facility.

Mother went through a long period of time when a large suction tube was put down her nose and into her throat. The tube was inserted to help keep Mother's lungs clear. At first it seemed like a good idea and she responded well. But when she continued to choke on fluids that built up in her lungs, it became harder to watch her be put through all that pain and torment for a temporary solution. I knew she would never want a ventilator or a feeding tube. However, the suction catheter used to clear her lungs was not so obvious a choice. She had to have secretions pulled out so she could breathe easier. At the last, as the suctioning became more frequent, and her body weakened, we knew she would not get better.

On her last visit to the emergency room from the health care facility, the doctor on call explained in detail aspiration pneumonia and said that she would just go through this again and again. He asked "Do you want us to proceed with the suction?" I was not prepared for the question. I had not considered that this was an option. It was hard to let go; she was old, tired, sick, and ready to die, yet she could still smile and hold my hand.

My immediate answer to him was "Yes." As I watched her discomfort as they put the tube in her nose, I wondered, "Why should she have to go through this again?" Later in ICU, the breathing mask was on, her hands bruised again from the many punctures to get the IV in, and her lungs were clearly filling with fluid. She coughed hard, her face reddened, her veins in her forehead looked as though they would pop, and I kept thinking, "This is not good."

Some would have let her go long ago. After all, what possible benefit is this little old lady to anyone? But they didn't see that twinkle in her eye; they didn't hear her sweet voice; however rattled it was; they didn't feel the tight squeeze on my hand. They could not know how much she meant to me or how my heart was breaking. "Lord, this is so very, very hard; help me never judge another in this position."

A nurse had told me long ago, you have to be an advocate for your mother. You must check and re-check and let people know when things are not right.

I'm too tired. I'm hurt and I'm scared. I don't want to be a strong patient advocate any more. I want Mommy to hold me in her arms and tell me every-

thing is going to be okay. I want the two of us to go home with Russell and sit by the fire and watch the birds at the birdfeeders until the sun goes down.

GOING HOME!

Little Robin with your head held so high, do you know my heart is breaking? Do you care at all? You strut your stuff so proudly and sing there among the tall grasses and dandelions. I can see you are chirping along, grabbing a bug to eat as you go. I'm almost mad at you for being so happy! Doesn't the whole world need to stop and feel my pain and hurt? How can life go on so normally around me while I'm here dying inside? Some would say you're here to cheer me up. Well, sorry little birdie, it's not working!

While watching my mother lay in that hospital bed perhaps taking her last breaths, it was so hard to enjoy the beauty of nature outside her window. In days past, she and I both would have marveled at God's great creation and enjoyed to the max the beautiful robins at play. How fickle I was when the waves hit so hard.

Mother celebrated her 90th birthday at home. Russell's sister, Nellie Beene's birthday was the same date so he had gone to Oklahoma to be with her, leaving Mother and I to enjoy the day together. It was a beautiful, sunny day. Mother had received dozens of cards which I stood up on her table. I sang "Happy Birthday" to her before she got out of bed. She looked happy as we cuddled and enjoyed the morning. She ate a good breakfast and enjoyed television before taking a nap. I spent lunchtime in her room with her; she ate most of her lunch all by herself. We watched the birds at the feeders outside her window and talked about how God had blessed us both. She was all smiles as I reminded her she was ninety years old.

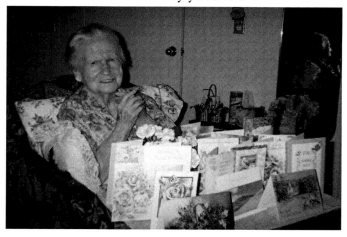

A few days after her birthday, she was taken to the emergency room and admitted to the hospital. Her big blue eyes were just little cold slits in her sad face as she looked at me as if to say, "Can't you fix me?" Even then she puckered for a kiss as the attendants wheeled her into the examining room.

A couple of weeks later, Mother was in the Intensive Care Unit of the hospital. She could hardly move, but she clung to my hand most of the day. I softly sang some old hymns to her like *Rock of Ages* and *Precious Memories.* For a little while, she sang with me in a tiny, tiny voice. I told her often that she could go home. "Mommy, if God has your home ready, you can go. It's okay if you go home. I love you."

Having the positive assurance of heaven made our expected parting so much easier. This reassurance was repeated several times before she actually went home. "Mommy, I'll keep you forever if you want me to; but, I'll let you go be with Jesus when you are ready."

As the days turned into weeks, then months, I began to feel the loneliness of her empty bedroom. How I wanted to go in to give her hugs; to check on her, and make sure she was okay. I didn't recall ever feeling so lonely and so helpless.

Early one Sunday morning, a physician called to say Mother was so much better. He gave her a stronger antibiotic and resumed some of her other medications and said they would move her to the floor from ICU soon. Because of his good report we were able to take time after church to have a relaxing meal and visit with friends.

Mother's ICU nurse was in the gift shop as we entered the hospital that afternoon. She beamed as she shared how well Mother was doing that morning. It was comforting to know that Mother would be finally in a room with a television to watch, pictures on the wall, and good surroundings to occupy her mind. ICU is a frightening place when you are well, and certainly so for an elderly, sick woman.

Mother had been moved out to the floor. However, as we approached her room, I began to feel uneasy. It did not appear to be a regular hospital room. We went through a small entry room into a larger room; her bed was at the far end with a small table on one side and a chair on the other. There was no television at all. The walls were dreary and bare.

We stopped frozen at the door. Mom's eyes were focused on us in a cold stare and her chest was really rattling. Right away we knew that the earlier good report was not as what we had anticipated, and we were crushed to find her in such a terrible state.

²"*Trust and obey, for there's no other way . . .*" The song ran through my head and I managed a cheerful smile as we approached her bed. Every part of my being wanted to run out of there, and cry. I wanted to find out why she was in a different kind of room. First, I had to let her know everything was okay. A nurse had caught me on the way into the room. "You must put on gloves and a gown before you enter." What mixed emotions I had! There is no way you can be prepared for these very different reports in the same hour.

Later the doctor on duty talked with me about her condition and the reason for the room. He explained she had Methacillian Resistant Staph Aureous

(MRSA), and she had to be isolated for a few days. She had to have chest x-rays and blood checks often, and they had to balance the very strong antibiotics.

I was told that, in hospital settings with so many chronically ill patients, staph infections are common. The difference in MRSA and other staph infections is its resistance to antibiotics. Because it is so difficult to treat, isolation becomes necessary. It would have relieved a lot of tension for me to have been told all this before I found her in that isolated room.

This scenario would play over and over again in one form or another for weeks. I soon came to realize that "good" was relative and that each "down" time would become harder and harder. While my inner struggle is impossible to explain, I think these journal entries express it best.

Tuesday, May 4, 2004

I'll never be prepared for the drastic up and downs of the process. I got here before 7:00 am; she's fast asleep and obviously pretty out of it. A nurse tries to revive her but to no avail. Doctor Evans came by on rounds and she looked at him, then to the ceiling. She did not look toward me at all, even with coaxing. The doctor talked with me about what was happening to her body. Then he took my hand and hers and had prayer, asking God to bless her, and thanking Him for her life. She went off to sleep. About 9:00 a.m. the nurse suctioned her lungs, and cleaned her mouth with a lemon swab.

She said I should go home and rest as there was nothing any of us could really do for her now. I chose to wait awhile before leaving.

Mother did rally a little and I gave her some cream of wheat and a little apple juice. She was able to focus on me as I fed her and then dropped off to deep sleep again; hands folded on her chest. It's 10:00 a.m. and I'm going home for a short time; not knowing what to expect on my next visit. At 4:00 p.m. Russell came with me to the hospital. I was thankful he would be with me whatever we faced as we walked into the room. Being prepared for the worst, I was again surprised at her condition.

The speech therapist, Mary Kuehmichel, was using some electrical stimulation on her cheeks. Mary fed her Ensure and grape juice at the same time and Mother was responding very well. She swallowed on command, all the while watching Mary. When she didn't swallow, Mary reached for the suction tube and Momma swallowed quickly while giving her a dirty look. Sometimes she smiled a little and answered, "uh, huh" or "no" in response to questions. Mary talks about how well she's doing and tells of the new goals for her. Just this morning the nurse had said we would hold off on any kind of therapy. I'm confused again, Lord. Only You know. Help my unbelief.

The therapy Mary used is called VitalStim Therapy, a relatively new procedure. The electrical stimulation lifts the larynx and strengthens the muscles around it. Because muscles get weaker with age, this has proven beneficial in prolonging life. Even someone Mother's age, with good health otherwise, can be helped immensely. Now I realize those "colds" I thought Mother kept getting may have been her aspirating. Here again, the doctor possibly could have helped earlier had he been more informed about her problems at home.

Several times during the last few weeks of her life, Mother found some words. One time she said she had a conversation with her mother. She began telling me all about it:

"I was talking with my mother."

"Was she here?"

"Yes."

"Everything okay?"

"She had to go."

"Did she go home?"

"She went home."

"Did she want you to go?"

"She wanted me to go home with her."

"Are you going to go?"

"No."

"You're not going?"

"No, not now."

I reassured her that, when she was ready to go be with her mother, it was all right with me, but that she didn't need to be in a hurry. We snuggled awhile and she drifted off to sleep. I was sure she was talking of heaven and was thankful she didn't want to go right now.

Another time she mumbled something about Butch (Richard) and Sue (me) and Frank (Dad) and the house being sheltered. She was talking about our family when my brother and I were small. I never did quite figure out what she was trying to say about the house being sheltered. Her expressions were positive so I knew it was not something that troubled her. It had been a good day for her; she had eaten well, and seemed quite content.

These were difficult weeks filled with ups and downs. Again my journal seems to describe those times best.

> *Some days I'm actually paralyzed just getting ready to go see her. I stand in the bathroom staring at my clothes and can't seem to move. All of a sudden I realize how much I don't want to go on this journey; I don't want my mother to go. I can stand by her bed and hold her hand and tell her it's okay. We can sing the songs and quote the scriptures as she looks into my eyes, but it's not okay. I don't want Mother to leave me. I need her. Sure, she can't do all the things she used to do, but I need her warm body to touch and to hold. I need her beautiful smile and that twinkle in her bright blue eyes. God, how can You ever fill this big, big hole in my heart?*

The emptiness leaves briefly as I listen to gospel music on the way to see her. But, as I near town, the loneliness comes back. Entering the hospital my feet are heavy. It's so hard to walk that long, long hall again, and I wonder how many more times will I do it?

Entering her room I see she's fast asleep and looking so peaceful. But my frozen heart just stops again. They've moved my chair! Her bed is in the middle of the room instead of to one side or another. There is no room to even move a chair over there. If I try to move the bed, that will surely wake her up. I'm so angry! I'm standing against the wall just watching her sleep and I am so cold inside. How does a broken heart keep breaking over and over again?

As she stirs, I move the bed and get the chair back in place. It always seemed so very, very important that I be really close to her when I was in the room. I took the mitt off her left hand; I don't think she will pull at her IV anymore. As I put lotion on her soft little hands and rub them gently, I think of the women preparing Jesus for burial. I know she will soon be with Him but it hurts so much to let her go.

It feels as if we are invisible as I watch the flurry of activity in the hallway. They wheel patients back and forth, some are walking with a nurse, medicines are being passed, and charts updated. Why can't someone help my mommy? We had prepared for everything and I thought I was prepared, too. But the finality of it all frightened me again. When the aides do come in her room they insist on opening all of her breakfast dishes and thickening all her liquids. Maybe it makes them feel better to do all they can. Aides and nurses come from other areas just to hug her and perhaps say "Good-bye." I look over all the "stuff" she would have to eat if she were better. She wouldn't choose to live like that and I can't choose it for her either. One nurse checked her heart rate and then left to crush her pills, and I wonder, 'What is the point?'

Days pass and she rallies again. She is awfully weak but quite alert. Her eyes watch every move I make, and she approves as I offer her a drink of juice. As I tilt the glass to give her a drink, she moves her fingers to take the glass and sip a little juice all by herself. Perhaps this will help her feel not so helpless and hopeless. I know that about one or two sips are all she will do and then fall to sleep, glass in hand. I'll take the glass and put it up. For this minute my mom can do some little something on her own. She needed it and so did I.

I spent as much time as possible with her. She couldn't express herself and I wanted to make sure she was cared for. More than that, I didn't want her to awaken and be frightened with none of us there to reassure her that she was okay.

The day came when Mother would make one final move. This one was to the nursing home in our town, and I knew in my heart it would be her last one. This time I would need to spend more time than ever with her, knowing each day could be the last.

I spent hours just holding her hand, patting her, kissing her and telling her how much I loved her. That is all I could do for her. She would twiddle her thumbs a bit and drift off to sleep. Some days, she wouldn't care to eat at all and I wondered what the point was in trying to force it. On Saturday before she died, she did eat half her supper and I actually got a smoochie! I can still feel that gentle touch and see that sweet face. Priceless memories!

At 1:30 a.m. on a Monday morning the nurse called to say Mother was not doing well. Russell rushed me to the nursing home. I appreciated him so much. He stayed for a short time and had prayer with us. Then he honored my request and went home. He loved Mother so much too; it was hard on him. He knew God had granted my prayer, and graciously allowed me this time with her. I had promised her many times that when her home was ready; I would be there to hold her hand until Jesus took it.

Hours passed slowly as I held her hand, and caressed her cool face. When I grew tired and tried to pull away, she would rally enough to hold on a little tighter. Her breathing was becoming quite heavy and her fingers were turning blue as her grip relaxed. She was so tired; every time she gasped a deep breath, I thought she was gone. The nurse brought me coffee and kept close watch on us. At one point, a nurse asked me if I wanted her to be taken to the hospital.

"No. No more hospitals for my mother. She has been through enough."

"Lord, take care of her; make her passing easy. She is so precious."

From the last journal entry:

> *As I observe the people in rooms and hallways, some are moaning and others rambling with unclear speech. Some are just out of it completely, some obviously in pain. I remember how blessed Mom has been. God in His grace has spared her much pain and confusion.*

> *At 6:00 am I run my finger over her hand, it's cold and still and blue. I recall all the work those hands have done in ninety years; good work and honorable. I think of all the care she's given to others. I think how much those who didn't get to know her have missed. I want her to go on home, but I miss her so much already.*

> *At 6:40 God answered my prayer. Mother peacefully went to sleep. No more pain. And I was blessed to be there holding her hand and singing to her, [3]'Blessed assurance, Jesus is mine! Oh, what a foretaste of glory divine! Heir of salvation, purchase of God, Born of His Spirit, washed in His blood.' 'Thank you, Jesus.'*

> *She has lost so much weight that her face looks*

more like the mom of my schooldays. She looks so peaceful and rested. All I can think of is the over-whelming goodness of God! What joy He has given me! Eight wonderful years of getting to love my mommy, and then get to participate in her home going. Oh, yes, God is good, heaven is real, and I am most blessed indeed.

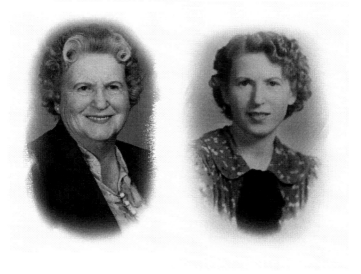

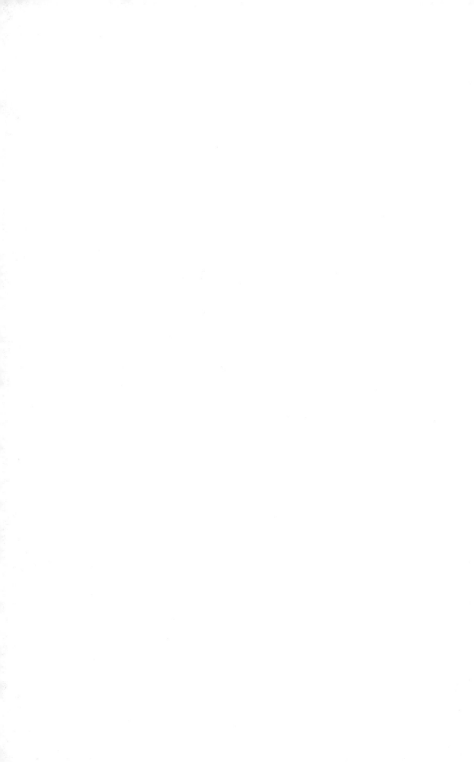

‿ᄋ

*M*other's death left a big hole in my heart; I miss her terribly. Life has changed drastically for me since she is gone. There are hours to fill that I didn't have when she was with us. There are also other losses that I had not anticipated.

Gone are the caregivers. Mary who had been in our home several times a week for seven years no longer comes. When she gave up the personal care and went to work at the hospital, we would still see her there; she continued to be like family as she took time each day to visit with Mother. Now she no longer comes by. She has new families who need her.

Gone are the friends from church who would come by often just to check on my Momma. Oh, they are still friends, and they still come by, but not like they did. After all, there are other folk who need them now, and they must move on with their lives, too. I praise

God for each of them, and the time they gave us so freely. I am quite sure their faithful prayers sustained us more than we will ever know.

Gone are some viewing habits we developed when Mother was with us. I miss the cartoons! She loved the happy scenes and the cheerful, lively music. A colorful animated show would come on and she would sit on the edge of her chair watching and laughing at the silly antics of some little bear or flower or whatever. It isn't really the cartoons that I miss; I miss watching her reaction to them. I also miss the laughter they brought into this house.

Something I never ever expected; gone are my excuses. You know, it was so easy if I didn't really want to go to a meeting or take part in a project to simply say that I should stay home with Mother. Everyone understood. It was a valid reason for not going. Now, I cannot use her as a crutch to get out of things. I must buckle up and do the things I know I should be doing with no excuses. This, too, is hard. Part of the difficulty was realizing how often I *had* used her without meaning to in some situations. As I said earlier, I am learning a lot about myself through this experience and it is not all easy.

If my house could talk, it would say it definitely misses Momma. It is obvious to those who visit that keeping house is not my main priority in life. Oh, it is always tidy and presentable at first glance; just don't check for dust or cobwebs. Those years with my mother watching me, I did do a better job of cleaning. And we had homemaker helpers that came in throughout the week. Cheryl Epps was one homemaker that kept our home shining, far better than I had ever done. She was thorough and fast. I miss that fresh, clean smell of a well-scrubbed home each week.

Cheryl was in the midst of cleaning the day the ambulance was called to take Mother to the hospital. I can still see her as she quietly gathered her things and left. I think she knew she would not come to our house again. She had grown to love Mother; it was evident in her constant concern for Mother's well-being. Cheryl was an outstanding worker and a caring, compassionate person. How hard that must be as caregivers see their clients slip away.

I think disposing of Mother's medications was the one of the hardest thing I've done. As I emptied the drawer, I had the deep sense she might need these things. Perhaps the difficulty was in the turning loose of this last responsibility. Every day I would prepare her pills and crush them and give them to her on time. There would be no more weekly calls to the physician or the pharmacy to check on one thing or another about her medicines.

I carefully cleared the bulk of personal items and clothing from her room. The wheelchair, walker, and rails from the hospital bed were neatly tucked away in the garage. When I gathered her fuzzy slippers from her shoe drawer I just cried. I held them tightly, remembering how hard it had been to find slippers for her. Later her feet and ankles slimmed down, and these shoes became way too big.

I folded the freshly washed towels and washcloths that had been used so many times in caring for Mother. As I worked, I looked up at the items on her wall and took time to watch the cows grazing in the field just beyond our fence. I could almost hear her proclaim, "I see the cows!" Joy quickly turned to sorrow as I realized that I would never hear that voice again. These clean linens would never be used to wash that precious face. Suddenly the pain was too real and too deep to express.

Mom and I had shared a big walk-in closet; now I will have it all to myself. I don't want the whole closet! I want to share it with my momma. I want to hang her things back up, to feel them and smell them. Closing my eyes, I can picture my precious little momma all dressed up in her new duds, waiting with a smile on her face for me to brag on how beautiful she looked.

In the care facility, they seemed to pack up Mother's clothes without a second thought; she was just another lady to them. They didn't know her, not really. How sad they only got to know the tired, old woman who was very, very ill. Oh, they loved her smiles, but they didn't know the vibrant woman she was.

I did keep a few tubs of her better things in the garage until I could find the best place to take them. Now I must clean it all out and take them someplace where they are needed. I wonder if down deep inside

I felt if I get rid of all her things, I'll be losing the memories, too. I can feel her softness in her clothes, smell her fragrance, and sense her being. Will it all fade away? I wonder . . .

Here is the little notebook I kept by her chair so she could make a grocery list for me. More than once I went to the store with a tiny page of scribbled lines or her list of interesting items such as "12 birds, 12 eggs, beads, candles, bunny rabbit, jumping jacks." "That looks like a pretty long list there," I would say as she handed me the book. "Did you miss anything? Want me to get some fruit, too?" The sweet smile and nod "Yes" are permanently imbedded in my memory; grocery shopping will never be the same.

What do I do with the notebook she scribbled in? And what about all these beautiful cards sent by family and friends through the years? You would know yellow roses were her favorite flower by all the silk ones scattered throughout her room and bathroom, but do I need them all now? These children's books with the corners chewed off aren't really any good for someone else. They are valued by me, but I cannot keep everything.

It was a few months after Momma died that I decided to clear out most of these "priceless" treasures. I chose a pretty wire basket and began to sort out the very best keepsakes: two well-chewed children's books, the small album of Enid, Oklahoma photographs, some envelopes she had used to practice writing her name, a few of her favorite cards and letters, my three favorite pictures of her, a well used tiny notebook, one yellow silk rose, and, of course, a baby book with rubber corners.

This is not meant to become a sacred basket or monument to her. Sitting proudly on the chest in "her" bathroom, it is merely a group of tender memories of treasured days gone by. The pretty basket serves as a gentle reminder of the child in each of us and the Faithful Father who unconditionally supplies our every need.

Momma's little hand reaches toward me and I feel her gently fingering all the buttons on my shirt as if checking to see if they are all intact. Then her hand straightens my collar. All the while her gaze seems to be on first my shirt and then me. "Are you checking me out? Am I all together. Is it okay?" That soft, gentle, approving smile says, "Yes."

I open my eyes, tears streaming down my cheeks and I feel if I just keep my eyes closed I can reach out and hug her.

But I can't . . .

Sometimes just walking into the store can bring tears. It just doesn't seem right to check out without getting Mother's bananas and her favorite cereal. In Wal-Mart I automatically go to the pharmacy first to check prices on Depends and other needed items. All those years of buying so many items for personal care and learning by trial and error which would work best gave me a wealth of knowledge. Now, I know more than I ever wanted to about things such as that, and no one needs them here.

> *So much has changed.*
> *No long shopping list,*
> *No protein drinks or special foods,*
> *No daily laundry to do,*
> *No Depends to buy,*
> *No box of detergent every week,*
> *No extra cleaning supplies,*
> *No disposable pads,*
> *No baby powder,*
> *No special soaps and creams,*
> *And, no Mommy!*

My eyes are scratchy and hurting; it feels as though there may be a hair in one of them. There is Visine in the medicine cabinet but when I reach for it, I remember all the times I would get that bottle down to use on Mom and I can't seem to take it from the cabinet. Will the reminders ever go away? What do I do with all this hurt?

One evening I decided to make something good and gooey for a snack. Russell and I had been eating healthy for quite a spell and I was aching for something better. All I could find in my kitchen was a box of sugar-free instant chocolate pudding. Well, chocolate is good! My conscious thoughts were on the busy-ness of the day and the desire for a snack. I grabbed a bowl and added the mix and milk. Closing the lid carefully I began to vigorously shake the mixture. And then the tears fell uncontrolled as my mind recalled Momma's delight when she knew I was going into the kitchen to make pudding. Almost in a trance the familiar images replayed before me; chopping up bananas for her pudding to add extra nutrition; fixing her bib and putting her pudding in a footed goblet that she could hold easily. What joy watching her as she savored every bite. This was followed by the big cleanup when she was finished. Her pudding was down her chin and bib and all over her fingers and hands. That precious chocolate covered little-girl smile is permanently imbedded in my mind.

Sometimes I hurt so much; the hole is big and no one else can fill it. I had trusted God through all those years to see me through. He was there, holding my hand, caring for each of us. And now I needed His presence even more as our lives must be adjusted again. Re-reading another journal page reminded me again how good and ever-present our Heavenly Father is.

On Saturday, June 5, Mother had been gone two weeks. I was missing her so much. Then, God provided.

> The woman was old and frail and seemed to be barely standing as she leaned upon her grocery cart. As I neared her on my way into the store, I could see she had unloaded a portion of her groceries. She was breathing heavy and looked so tired. She looked up, 'I'm just tired' she said with labored voice. 'This was too much for me.'

I smiled and encouraged her to get in the front seat and let me do it for her. She got a banana from the cart and slowly made her way around the open back door to the front. Her labored steps affirmed she really was in trouble. As I finished the cart and closed the door, she looked better already.

'Are you okay now?' She nodded.

'Well, see now, I have a cart,' I replied.

'"It's a good one' she said.

'"I know it is; it was just used by a lovely lady.'

Her joy was apparent as I went on my way. My day had been a very rough one. I had gone to a Woman's Brunch at Urbana and then stopped by Enid's to cry with her. We both miss Mom so much. I then stopped at a sale or two on the way home. The emptiness just would not go away no matter what I did; seemed something was missing.

That is when I had found myself in the store parking lot where I met the lady in trouble.

Now, inside the store, I have such peace and joy and purpose. I am enthusiastically shopping away, quietly singing as I go. God knew my heart and knew my need: today my greatest need had been just to have someone to care for again!"

A LETTER TO MOTHER

◦

*T*he many conversations that I didn't have with my mother are impossible now. There is much I would like to have explored, including her past, and mine. I wonder about her feelings, and her hopes and dreams. She could tell me why she made some of her choices in life. We could laugh, and cry, and share some special times together.

The conversations I long to have are just with my mother; not with the outside world. Some questions are too deep and too personal to share, private thoughts between a mother and a daughter. These will remain with me forever, not meant for anyone but her.

I visit with Momma in my mind and my heart quite often; I suppose she will always be close to me in that way. I would like to share one of those conversations with you. In doing so, I hope you will come to know God, Mother, and me a little better. My prayer is that you will be encouraged to *make time in your own life to visit with your loved ones before that door closes forever.*

If that door has already closed, consider writing a letter to that person anyway. Just pen every word you would like to say; every single word, good or bad. A friend just shared that she writes a letter to her mother every year. Her mother died five years ago, but writing to her helps my friend release those feelings hidden deep inside. Sometimes the letter is tear-stained by the time she is finished writing it.

❧

Dear Momma,

How did God pour so much sweetness and love into one little lady? Why did He let me be your daughter? You certainly are such a precious treasure.

I am not the only one who believes you are a beautiful person. Do you remember the many times I would tell you about my classmates saying how pretty you were? You always had the same reply, "That is so ridiculous. I am not pretty!"

Oh, but you were. Even when you came home from working all day in a hot kitchen, your hair was combed neatly, and you had taken time to put on lipstick. I always wished for your wavy red hair; you wished it were different. Isn't that the way we silly girls are?

I didn't listen as I should have to your tales of childhood. I recall you didn't seem to have had much of one. You were just thirteen when your dad died and you had to quit school to take care of your mother. That little mining community around Carl Junction, Missouri, could not have offered many opportunities for a young girl to earn money. How did you live? What kind of work did you do?

Your mother was sick often, you said. What was wrong with her? Did she ever work outside the home? She was such a good cook; I bet you learned a lot from her. I remember some of her unusual dishes like vinegar pudding and watermelon preserves. When I think of how you must have grown up, I can understand how you learned to feed our family of four those great feasts on practically nothing. If we had company drop in today, I would have to go to the store. You would probably be able to whip up a full meal, including dessert, from what is in my kitchen now!

What was life like when you were at home with your brother and sister? What were your pastimes? Did you go to church? Did Grandma make your clothes like you made ours when we were young?

When your brother, Virgil, was hit in the head with a baseball and died at the age of thirteen, was someone there to help you get through that? How terribly sad that must have been. And, where did you live when your sister, Josephine, received third degree burns from flames pouring out of a stove? Were you living close enough to help care for her? That must have been terrible for you both.

Later, when you and Aunt Josie both had lost little children of your own, life sounds unbearable. I don't even know what happened to the children; how they died, how old they were. Those difficult years must have been so painful. I wish we had talked more about those times in your life; and about Aunt Josie and her family.

Teenage years are troublesome at times, regardless of the era. I don't recall you talking much at all about your teen years. You were so very strict with my brother and me growing up; I think you must have had some difficult times yourself. Did you get to finish any of your schooling? If you didn't, you sure learned a lot on your own. I always thought you were so smart. I remember you taught us to read when we were very young; it was so important to you that we had an education.

You did talk often about your experiences when you were in your late twenties. I wish I knew how you became a governess in Oklahoma, and why you left. It sounds like such a special time in your life.

I have the poems you wrote in your twenties. They are good. Did you ever try to publish any of them? Did you share them with anyone or simply keep the original copies for yourself?

You said one time that you dated a Baptist preacher. How ironic that I should eventually end up married to one. Momma, I sure wish you could tell me about your preacher boy friend. You would have been a great pastor's wife; you are so supportive and strong. I am curious, too, about your faith. Jesus must have been very real to you at a young age. You went through so much as a child and young adult; He had to be with you each step of the way.

In sorting through some more papers today, I found a Cosmetology and Hairdressing Certificate dated 1940, from The State Board of Health of Missouri. It certifies that Katie Geneva Phillips completed a course in cosmetology and hairdressing, including manicuring. It does not say where the license was issued. I wonder where you were living when you took this course.

One time when we visited Lanagan, you showed me where your beauty shop had been before it burned with everything in it. I am so thankful you kept your license somewhere safe; it gives me another glimpse of your life. No wonder I had the prettiest hair in school (although I didn't always appreciate it at the time). You gave permanents to half my classmates and their mothers, often after coming home from a long, hard day at work. Where did you get your energy?

All I recall about you and Daddy dating is that you said, "He was sure handsome in that Army outfit!" Where and how did you meet? I would like to hear all the juicy details of your courtship. I know the war cut your plans short; soon you were married, and there I was.

Were you glad I came? Was I a surprise? I'm

glad you kept me! When did we move way back into the woods on acreage behind Dad's folks' house? There you were with absolutely no utilities in the house and two babies to care for. I would like to know what the little house looked like. You had to carry all of the water up from the bottom of the hill. How did you manage to keep us all clean?

I wish you would have told me more about the short time we were in California, where I started to kindergarten. In my memory bank, there is a time when I was under a table on a lawn with some friends. I can close my eyes and smell the freshly cut grass and see the flowers blooming profusely. I'd like to know if it was on an army base, or in a friend's yard. I was only four or five, but I remember our lives were so happy then. You said we moved back to Missouri to take care of your parents, and Dad's. I doubt if you really wanted to move.

All my childhood years, I watched you care for elderly parents as best you could. With just a two-room home of our own, we could not take them in. But, after you worked hard six or seven days a week, you found time to take them shopping and tend to their needs as well. Daddy's parents lived about an hour away in one direction and yours that far in the other direction. Didn't you ever just want to give up?

Now that I think about it, your time seemed to just stretch more than most. When we were in school, you took time to help us with lessons. You went to PTA meetings to see how we were doing and how you might help. Remember that time you decided we needed a park in Goodman? I can still see you talking with all who would listen and, as I recall, we cleaned off some property for one. I wonder if that land is still being used for a park.

One of my fondest memories is of you playing basketball. I don't know how the team even got started or why you joined. I can still see your serious expression when you got the ball in your possession. We could spend much time here, so much I would like to hear you talk about. Why didn't we share those moments when we could?

When and how did you find time to be our 4-H Community Leader? You were a good one. Everyone loved my momma. You just had a way about you that drew people to you. The up and up, and the down and out; they all respected you.

Remember when Richard and I would get sick and you made us clay to play with? I didn't ever get the recipe. Oh, there are recipes for home-made clay around; I've seen many of them. But none of them compare to yours. It was just the right consistency to build great figures, and the colors were perfect. I suppose, Mother, it was really not the recipe that made that clay so good. It was just right because you made it for us.

Where did you learn how to do so much? You didn't just teach us to make tissue mums or crepe-paper roses. We learned to make all sorts of beautiful flowers from paper. You sewed so well, by hand, or on the machine. You taught us to sew as well. Richard and I each embroidered a pillowcase with deer on it. Maybe that is why I am so attracted to the deer in our meadow.

You really enjoyed being a mother and home-maker. I could tell by the way you kept our tiny home. Everything had a place and we didn't dare leave our things strung around the house. We had our chores to do, and you made sure we did them right. I was not so happy with you when you made me dust again because I didn't put fresh scarves on the dresser and chest. Of course, now I am glad you taught me to do things correctly and didn't let me be lazy about my work.

Thanks for encouraging me to read and to draw. I think the way you appreciated each little thing we made for you was so great. No matter how busy or tired you were, you made time to admire our handi-work. You always bragged on Richard's flowers he grew for 4-H projects and the furniture he built. He got lots of ribbons at our county 4-H meetings and so did I. For cooking and sewing! No one would believe it now; but I still have proof!

Speaking of cooking, I have to say again that you were good! Your meatloaf, fried chicken, pork chops and gravy, and those big, fat biscuits. How I would like a plate of them now. I never, ever heard you say, "I'm so tired. Let's just have a sandwich tonight or go get a hamburger." Feeding your family warm, nutritious meals was more important to you than resting a spell. I would like to know how you canned those green beans and okra from our garden. No one's canning tastes like yours did. I can almost hear you saying, "You are so silly!" You never did like bragging, did you?

In the world's eye, we were poor folk. We just didn't know it. You made sure we knew we were as good as anyone. Material things did not have priority in your life and you helped Richard and I understand what was really important.

You taught me to love God and nature as we took our Saturday outings. Those trips were so special to me. I can still remember the excitement in your face when we rode the train at Silver Dollar City or viewed the peonies at the Sarcoxie nurseries. You always mentioned the 'beautiful world that God made.' There was no question in my mind who is the Creator of the universe.

We could tell that you and Dad loved each other so much. You pampered him like you taught us to do with our mates; and sometimes, he gave back to you. You both were so good to your ailing parents, never complaining or refusing to help them when they needed you.

It was fun when we all went to the woods to pick huckleberries and blackberries. You would get so mad when Daddy would sneak off and find the biggest berries to quickly fill his bucket. Even then, you could out pick him!

But he was a rascal, Momma. How did you ever put up with his drinking and chewing that old Copenhagen? You were always so neat and tidy. He was, too, sometimes. But when he got on a drinking spell, he was a mess! You never condemned him to us and wouldn't let us talk about him either. Night after night, when he didn't come home for supper on time, you would still leave him a big, warm plate of good food to eat.

Some of those years were hard on all of us. I suppose you could not have left if you had wanted to. After all, where would you go with two little ones in tow? And, as I said, I know you loved him. In a more private conversation, I have so much I would like to ask you about. So many unanswered questions; so many things I want to tell you, but never did. Some things may be better off left unsaid, at least for now.

I know things got so much better for you when you quit work and you and Daddy had a bigger house. No longer drinking, he did a good job of providing for you. You had Richard's son, Andy, to care for while his parents worked. Dad had his gardening and working on the rental houses. You two could now enjoy your senior years together.

What a tragedy when Daddy took his life. I remember that look of horror on your face when we found him. Having to call my brother and tell him what had happened was so hard. Those nights I awakened to hear you crying were almost unbearable. I would go back there now if I could, and try to comfort you. I would spend more time with you in the day talking through all the thoughts we both shared. I would want to let you know it wasn't something you did or didn't do. Not that you don't know already, I just would want to say it to you. I wouldn't just pretend it didn't happen without talking about it. We will never understand why he chose to do it, especially when you were both doing so well. It would have helped us all to talk about it a little more openly.

Then, two years later, my husband died suddenly of a heart attack. There we were, two widows. You were so good to me and so patient. You always had the right things to say at the right time. And you took time for me when I was hurting.

After we adjusted to our plight, we had fun, didn't we? The world was ours and we could go anywhere and do anything we wanted (within our small budgets). We were ladies on the move. Church, Bible studies, painting classes, art shows; we were ready for any opportunity to learn something new.

That's when we met my Baptist preacher. Only God could have orchestrated the events that led us to join the church Russell pastored. When we joined Harmony Heights Baptist Church in Joplin, we had no idea what God had in store. I married the preacher and you got really involved in their single adult class. Practically overnight, we both had plenty of new friends and a church that could use our time and talents.

Momma, do you remember those hours we spent making beautiful feather mums and gladiolas for my wedding? That horrible blizzard almost closed the roads, but we made it to church on wedding day. Did you wonder about your daughter through all that time, or had you prayed for such a time as that? Could you ever imagine that in twenty years, that preacher would be helping take care of you? I think we're both glad "we" married him!

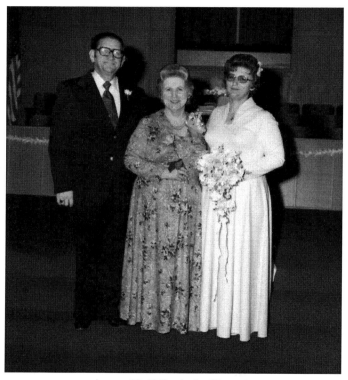

January 13, 1979   Joplin, Missouri

I would sure like to know more about your faith. You were always so morally good, and made sure my brother and I went to church. You'd be surprised, Momma, to know the lives you touched by your quiet steadfastness. I'm so proud of you. Your gentle faith

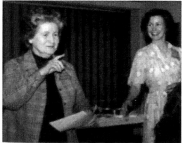

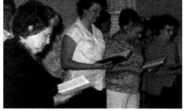

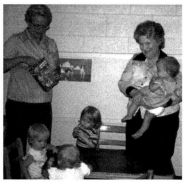

influenced others to be kinder, too.

I will never forget the day in LIFT Class (ladies' Bible study) when I asked the ladies to give a favorite Bible verse. I was shocked when you were the first to stand, and you quoted I John 5:14–15 without missing a word. I can almost hear your confident voice now.

And this is the confidence that we have in him, that, if we ask any thing according to his will, he heareth us: And if we know that he hear us, whatsoever we ask, we know that we have the petitions that we desired of him. KJV

When you quoted those verses that day, I began to recognize where you got all your strength. Your hope was in Jesus! We somehow grew closer after that; not just mother and daughter, but now real sisters in Christ.

When did you learn those verses? Was it from

your parents or Sunday School? I don't know if you went to church as a child. Your mother used to ask me to read the Bible to her when we were at her house, so I know God's Word was very comforting to her. The Bible was not that important to me at the time, and I read it just to please her. Oh, Momma, such treasured times I missed with you both.

In the 16th chapter of I Samuel, God tells Samuel that, ". . . man looketh on the outward appearance, but the Lord looketh on the heart." KJV Mother, I just know that God loved your pure heart. I often hear women share their love for God, and how He was with them in trying times. I wish we would have talked more about God at work in your life. Those stories of how He held your hand through rough times would mean so much to me now.

Did you ever give any thought to what God had planned for your life? You wrote some good poems; painted some beautiful pictures; taught a great Bible lesson; and could tend those babies in the nursery with ease.

I want to know what you wanted to be when you grew up. Did the demands of everyday life just carry you away from your dreams? You could have been a great writer or composer or artist. Perhaps even a skilled children's worker. You earned wages as a laundry worker, dinner cook, baker, governess, and later as a beautician. While you excelled at all you did, I think your real calling was to be a mother and a wife; you were very good at both. I do wonder, though, if circumstances had been different for you, what you might have felt led to pursue. I want to sit down by your side and hear you talk of all these things.

We could begin with these big photo albums I'm looking through now. Here is a cute picture of you as a child. Who is that with you? It doesn't look like Grandma. I don't know very many of these people. As you carefully placed each picture in the album, I know it brought back many memories. The worn pages tell me you enjoyed looking at them again and again. It is regrettable that the pictures are not dated and there are no names written down. Precious memories are gone forever. This album that meant so much to you is now sadly put away; its secrets forever sealed within.

I want to know about my growing up years; so much I don't remember. There are so many things I would like to tell you about, too. And, there are many things I still don't want to tell you. I'm sure you never told your mother everything you did either! I guess there are some things better left untold.

I was such an ornery squirrel. I wonder how many of your quiet prayers sustained me through life. Your mother spent many hours on her aching knees at the foot of her old feather bed. She prayed aloud for an hour every night. She didn't leave any of us out. I never saw you on your knees literally. I know now that your heart must have been on its knees twenty-four hours a day for you and your family.

There is so much more I want to ask you. So much I want to tell, but time has passed for such as that. It doesn't really matter now, does it? All these things I want to talk about simply pale in contrast to where you are now.

You could probably quote the words of Jesus in John 14.

> *Let not your heart be troubled: ye believe in God, believe also in me. In my Father's house are many mansions: If it were not so, I would have told you. I go to prepare a place for you. And if I go and prepare a place for you, I will come again, and receive you unto myself: that where I am there ye may be also. KJV*

And, He did come for you, just as He promised. The best moment for me in all of life was holding your hand, knowing Jesus would take it and escort you to your new home.

What a reunion there must have been in heaven when you saw your mother and your father, your sister and your brother. All those loved ones who had accepted Christ's sacrifice on the cross and His forgiveness of sins were there. Wow!

I know you walked straight and tall down those golden streets with Jesus. Someday, I'll be there, too. We will walk hand in hand together, and have eternity to talk. I don't think all these lost conversations will matter then, do you, Mother?

I think we will just worship God and be at peace.

Oh, what a day that will be!

Your loving daughter,

Sue

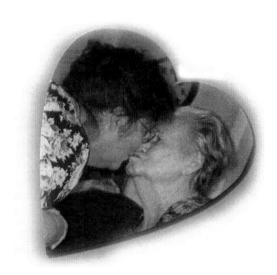

"I love you, Mommy!"

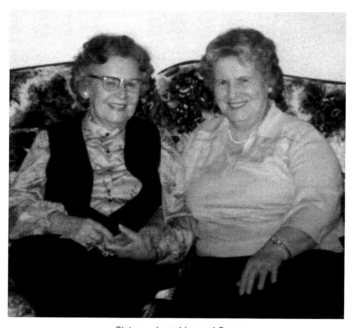

Sisters - Josephine and Geneva

TO OUR DARLINGS
By Katie Geneva Phillips–October, 1933

Just two little rays of sunshine
Were Grace and Pat, our babes so dear.
They were sent from God in Heaven
To encourage and to cheer.
Inspiring our hopes for things far better,
Teaching us of a brighter way,
Helping us to realize the blessings
We are enjoying every day.
Just a little while they stayed here,
But, oh! We shall never forget
The holy brightness of their presence
We know they were Heaven sent.
We cannot resent their going
Though we miss our babies dear.
For we too shall be called to Heaven
We shall meet again up there.

Written for her sister, Josephine Durfey Harry, after the
death of Josephine's two children.

HELPFUL SCRIPTURES

⟳

"I waited patiently for God to help me; then he listened and heard my cry" (Psalm 40:1, TLB).

"Don't worry about anything; instead, pray about everything; tell God your needs and don't forget to thank him for his answers. If you do this you will experience God's peace, which is far more wonderful than the human mind can understand. His peace will keep your thoughts and your hearts quiet and at rest as you trust in Christ Jesus" (Philippians 4:6–7, TLB).

"Thou wilt keep him in perfect peace, whose mind is stayed on thee: because he trusteth in thee" (Isaiah 26:3, KJV).

"And let the peace of God rule in your hearts . . . and be ye thankful (Colossians 3:15, KJV).

"And whatsoever ye do in word or deed, do all in the

name of the Lord Jesus, giving thanks to God and the Father by him (Colossians 3:17, KJV).

" . . . is your life full of difficulties and temptations? Then be happy, for when the way is rough, your patience has a chance to grow. So let it grow . . . when your patience is finally in full bloom, then you will be ready for anything, strong in character, full and complete" (James 1:2–4, TLB).

"Come unto me, all ye that labour and are heaven laden, and I will give you rest. Take my yoke upon you, and learn of me; for I am meek and lowly in heart: and ye shall find rest unto your souls. For my yoke is easy, and my burden is light" (Matthew 11:28–30, KJV).

"I can do all things through Christ which strengtheneth me" (Philippians 4:13, KJV).

"Because the Lord is my Shepherd, I have everything I need! He lets me rest in the meadow grass and leads me beside the quiet streams. He gives me new strength. He helps me do what honors him the most." (Psalm 23:1–3, TLB).

"I will praise thee, O Lord, with my whole heart; I will shew forth all thy marvelous works" (Psalm 9:1–2, KJV).

"I had fainted, unless I had believed to see the goodness of the Lord in the land of the living. Wait on the Lord, be of good courage, and he shall strength thine heart: wait, I say, on the Lord" (Psalm 27:13–14, KJV).

"I will bless the Lord who counsels me; he gives me wisdom in the night. He tells me what to do" (Psalm 16:7, TLB).

"But I am trusting you, O Lord. I said, 'you alone are my God, my times are in your hands'" (Psalm 31:14, 15a, KJV).

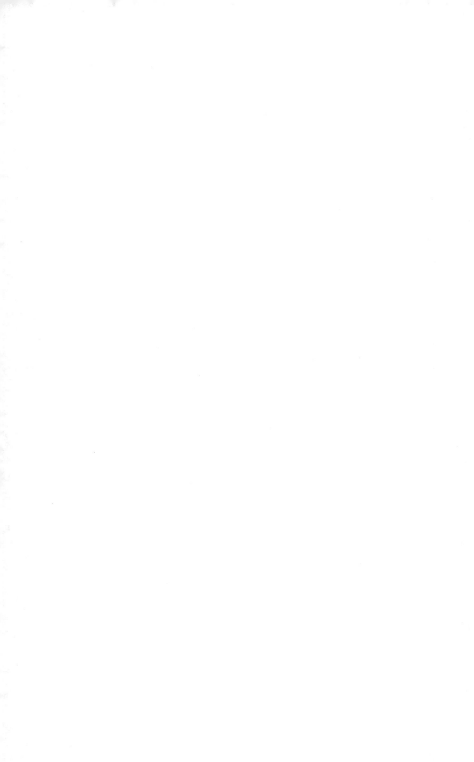

BOOKS

Barbara Deane, *Caring For Your Aging Parents, When Love is Not Enough.* Colorado Springs, CO: NavPress, 1989.

Henry Holstege, Ph.D. and Robert Rieskse, Ph.D, *Complete Guide to Caring for Aging Loved Ones.* (The official book of the Focus on the Family Physicians Resource Council). Wheaton, IL: Tyndale House Publishers, Inc., 2002.

WHERE TO FIND HELP

Local Church and Ministerial Alliance: When searching for home healthcare workers I found these two venues quite helpful. Many people in local churches have had need of such help and can provide references for people they might have worked with. Several communities offer information and resources through their local Ministerial Alliance; the telephone directory is a good place to begin your search.

Doctors and Hospitals: Because they are concerned for the total well being of the patient, they often can refer you to available programs that can help you in caring for your loved one.

Department of Health and Social Services, Division of Aging, Department of Human Resources, or Senior Citizens' Service Organizations: See local and state listings in the telephone directory.

Telephone Book: See listings under Health Care Facilities, Home Health Services, Hospices, Hospital Equipment & Supplies-Retail.

State Ombudsman Programs: Most states have an ombudsman program to investigate complaints by the elderly on conditions in nursing homes or adult-care-homes. Check the telephone directory for your State Ombudsman Program.

RESOURCE DIRECTORY

⎯⎯

Administration on Aging (AoA), 330 Independence
Avenue SW, Washington, D.C. 20201, 202-
619–7501 (National Aging Information Center),
800–677–1116 (Eldercare Locator), Web s i t e :
http://www.aoa.gov
The AoA, an agency of the U.S. Department of
Health and Human Services, educates   o l d e r
people and caregivers about the benefits and services available to help them.

American Geriatrics Society Foundation for Health in
Aging, 350 Fifth Avenue, Suite 801, New Y o r k ,
NY 10018, 212–308–1414, Web site: http://www.
healthinaging.org
AGS's foundation provides an aging-information
clearinghouse and an online manual   c a l l e d
Eldercare at Home.

American Health Care Association Publications, P. O. Box 3161, Frederick, MD 21705–3161, 800–628–8140, Web Site: http://www.ahca.org
The AHCA offers a free consumer's guide to nursing facilities and publications about nursing homes, guardianship, assisted living, finances, and long-term-care services.

Assisted Living Federation of America (ALFA), 11200 Waples Mill Road, Suite 150, Fairfax, VA 22030, 703–691–8100, Web site: http://www.alfa.org
ALFA provides publications and an on-line directory for locating an assisted living residence in your area.

BenefitsCheck*Up*, Web site: http://www.benefits-checkup.org
Free, on-line service identifies federal and state assistance programs for older Americans in all 50 states. Created to serve older adults who are eligible for benefits but do not know how to apply for them.

Caregiving.com/Caregiving Newsletter, P. O. Box 224, Park Ridge, IL 60068, 847–823–0639, W e b site: http://www.caregiving.com
This on-line resource and monthly print publication help persons who are caring for an a g i n g relative.

Children of Aging Parents (CAPS), 1609 Woodbourne
Road, Suite 302A, Levittown, PA 19057, 8 0 0–
227–7294, Web site: http://www.caps4caregivers.
org
CAPS is a national, nonprofit referral-and-re-
source information organization dedicated to
caregivers of the elderly, covering all aspects of
caregiving.

Christian Caregivers, P. O. Box 2573, Elk Grove, CA
95759–2573, Web site: http://www.Christian-
caregivers.com
Christian Caregivers provides information and
resources for caregivers and their families, including information about starting a caregiving ministry at church.

Geriatric Resources, Inc., P. O. Box 239, Radium
Springs, NM 88054, 800–359–0390 or 505-
524–0250, Web site: http://www.geriatric-resourc-
es.com
This company specializes in Alzheimer's caregiving
resources and services.

Home Health Equipment and Supplies by Mail: www.
exmed.net
Full line of home health supplies and equipment
including hard-to-find items. Ask for catalog for
mail order or a   list of stores near you that carry
specific product lines.

Incontinence Products: HDIS 800–844–2352.
Call for free catalogue and coupons. If you are not sure exactly what brand you prefer or the size you need, they have packages of samples to help with those decisions.

National Association for Continence, P. O. Box 8310, Spartanburg, SC 29305–8310, 864–579- 7 9 0 0 or 800-BLADDER (252–3337), Web site: http:// www.nafc.org
This not-for-profit organization offers a newsletter and products designed to improve the   quality of life of people with incontinence.

National Association for Home Care (NAHC), 228 7th Street, S.E., Washington, D.C. 20003,   202–547–7427, Web site: http://www.nahc.org
NAHC's Web site offers a free consumer guide on how to choose a home-care provider.

Perineal/Skin Care and Ostomy Products: Convatec 800–422–8811.

VitalStim Therapy: 1–800–506–1130.
www.vitalstimtherapy.com Information on treatment for people who have difficulty swallowing. Webmaster@ChattGroup.com Information on neuromuscular electrical stimulation used to treat dysphagia.

Well Spouse Foundation, 30 East 40th Street, New
    York, NY 10016, 800–838–0879, Web site:
    http://www.wellspouse.org
    This national, not-for-profit organization gives
    support to husbands, wives, and partners of the
    chronically ill and/or disabled.

(F O O T N O T E S)

⤸

[1] John Newton 1725–1807, arr. Edwin O. Excell 1851–1921, *Amazing Grace! How Sweet the Sound,* The Baptist Hymnal 1991, Convention Press

[2] John H. Sammis 1846–1919, Daniel B. Towner 1850–1919, *Trust and Obey,* The Baptist Hymnal 1991, Convention Press.

[3] Fanny J. Crosby 1820–1915, *Blessed Assurance, Jesus Is Mine,* The Baptist Hymnal 1991, Convention Press

To Contact the Author:

Please visit her website at:

www.susiekinslowadams.com

Or email:

info@susiekinslowadams.com

susie@susiekinslowadams.com

or order more copies of this book at:

TATE PUBLISHING, LLC

127 East Trade Center Terrace
Mustang, Oklahoma 73064

(888) 361 - 9473

TATE PUBLISHING, LLC
www.tatepublishing.com